# Creating Space

*Story, Reflection and Practice in
Healthcare Chaplaincy*

— SACHA PEARCE & JAN COLLIS —

Sacristy
Press

**Sacristy Press**
PO Box 612, Durham, DH1 9HT

www.sacristy.co.uk

First published in 2022 by Sacristy Press, Durham

Copyright © Sacha Pearce & Jan Collis 2022
The moral rights of the authors have been asserted.

All rights reserved, no part of this publication may be reproduced or transmitted in any form or by any means, electronic, mechanical photocopying, documentary, film or in any other format without prior written permission of the publisher.

Scripture quotations, unless otherwise stated, are from the New Revised Standard Version Bible: Anglicized Edition, copyright © 1989, 1995 National Council of the Churches of Christ in the United States of America. Used by permission. All rights reserved worldwide.

Every reasonable effort has been made to trace the copyright holders of material reproduced in this book, but if any have been inadvertently overlooked the publisher would be glad to hear from them.

Sacristy Limited, registered in England & Wales, number 7565667

**British Library Cataloguing-in-Publication Data**
A catalogue record for the book is available from the British Library

ISBN 978-1-78959-213-9

# Contents

**Acknowledgements** .................................................. iv

Chapter 1. A story of healthcare chaplaincy ....................... 1
Chapter 2. Defining practical theology ........................... 26
Chapter 3. Reflective practice: chaplain research in healthcare ...... 31
Chapter 4. What does "being" look like? .......................... 62
Chapter 5. Creating Space: The Pastoral Encounter ............... 79
Chapter 6. Conferences—teaching and nourishing a wider team ... 100
Chapter 7. Sharing "learning from discoveries" ................... 108
Chapter 8. Finding a chaplain: discernment—what does a
    chaplain look like? .......................................... 118
Chapter 9. Living with a virus ................................... 139
Chapter 10. Looking back and looking forward .................. 162

**Bibliography** ................................................... 174

# Acknowledgements

Our story, unfolding through reflection and developing practice, can only have developed with the support of a number of people both inside and outside the hospital environment. In a way, though, our acknowledgements begin and end with the staff of University Hospitals Plymouth at Derriford, including the ongoing support of the hospital Trust, Chief Executive Ann James, and the senior staff and nursing management.

This story began with the help of the healthcare professionals who have been involved in the research into reflective practice for wellbeing, giving space to reflect with a chaplain, learning together and giving each other a voice. Their continued day-to-day company, walking with them as individuals and/or as a team, on a regular basis or in response to an event, is a total privilege and a source of significant discovery.

During the early days and every day since, our evolving story would have been impossible without the contribution, energy and insight of our team, the Department of Pastoral and Spiritual Care, our fellow chaplains and pastoral visitors. We have learnt to give each other space, to listen to one another and share in the great adventure for learning. We celebrate that, both anonymously and unwittingly, every patient in every pastoral encounter has given us such rich material from which to learn and develop. We have also gained so much from our students on placement; the multidisciplinary nature of those taking our pastoral care training course; and the company of our wayfarers, those who have joined our community for a period of time and then stepped away, continuing their own journey. We thank, too, our chaplaincy colleagues in the South West for supporting us as we have shared our discoveries with them.

Working in both practical and public theology, we celebrate our vocation to accompany those in places of acute human experience, meaning our work as healthcare chaplains, licensed and supported here by the Anglican Church. We thank Bishop Sarah Mullally for her enthusiasm for our work and pastoral training while she was Bishop of Crediton, and also for inviting us to share our story with the Diocese of Exeter. We give our sincere thanks to the senior diocesan staff for their ongoing recognition of our work as the role of the chaplain increases in visibility.

Our thanks are offered to Dr Natalie Watson and Sacristy Press for believing that our story should be told and helping us share it.

Thank you to family and friends who have read chapters, commented on the project and generally listened to us too!

In our acknowledegment of all who have journeyed with us, we return to where we started in our incalculable thanks to the staff and management of Derriford Hospital and University Hospitals Plymouth NHS Trust for working with us and believing in our contribution to the life and wellbeing of this hospital and beyond.

May *your* story inspire reflections that bring you a wealth of discovery in your own practice!

CHAPTER 1

# A story of healthcare chaplaincy

*Creating Space* tells a professional and personal story of healthcare chaplaincy. It models the contextual storytelling and practice development of practical theology. By taking time, creating space for reflection, this book also reveals to healthcare, the Church and the community, the unique role of the chaplain and our experiences as a resource to others. We open the door outwards, inviting those both inside and outside the hospital to hear us reflecting on our process of developing and modelling our practice. We open the door to offer space for our story to inspire others to reflect on theirs, in their own context. This is our story of healthcare chaplaincy in context of over ten years of practice, in a team of chaplains in a hospital in the south-west of England.

University Hospitals Plymouth NHS Trust (UHPNT) runs the largest hospital in the peninsula, Derriford Hospital, which opened in 1981 and delivers a full range of general hospital services to people living in Plymouth, south and west Devon and Cornwall at a number of sites across the city and counties. As a specialist hospital, it operates at the heart of the south-west peninsula providing specialist hospital services within a wider peninsula population of more than 1.5 million. It is a teaching hospital in partnership with the University of Plymouth, and also works with Plymouth Marjon University. As host to the South West Medical Defence Group in a city with a strong military tradition, there is a tri-service staff of two hundred-plus military doctors, nurses and allied health professionals fully integrated within the hospital workplace. UHPNT serves a diverse population with a wide variation in health and life expectancy, within which there are pockets of deprivation. More than 48,000 people pass through the main entrance of Derriford Hospital each week, without taking into account the other entrances or indeed other centres. Derriford Hospital has just over 900 beds in thirty-six wards, of which 167 are day-case beds, and forty-one are for children. In 2019/20, 128,000 patients were cared for on the wards, there were 518,000 out-patient appointments and 142,000 emergency attendances. UHPNT employs close to 8,500 people.

Derriford's five chaplains (whole time equivalent) together with almost a hundred volunteers, work in the Department of Pastoral and Spiritual Care to provide pastoral, spiritual and religious support to patients, staff and visitors. For this team, creating space means making room for a story to be heard and for practice to evolve. Here there is an adventure for learning, inspiring chaplains and their team to reveal how they are learning from their experiences.

*Creating Space* is a story that shares our discoveries and makes them accessible to others. It may be a handbook to be read cover to cover or else dipped into depending on the reader's context and interest. Each chapter or section shares our experiences and encourages others to consider how any of our discoveries may be helpful to them. This is a book for professional practitioners, prompting their own contextual learning and development, whether as chaplains, pastoral carers, parish clergy, lay ministers, volunteers in any caring context, those who work in listening therapies, those who provide care and support to others of any kind, or those who use or teach reflective practice.

Chapter by chapter, we reveal our story and the way in which each of our experiences is a source of learning. Outlining the highlights of the last ten years, we begin the story by looking through the lens of our own professional background and developing our understanding of the unique role of the healthcare chaplain, continuing to cultivate this with our model of "creating space". We connect in a straightforward way our view of healthcare chaplaincy as a model of practical theology, based on key practical theologians who see the human story as a source of learning. Drawing from this we describe our practical theology as being always willing to learn. We outline our own reflective practice tool for learning, and we share the way in which we see each pastoral encounter as a reflective source of learning. We demonstrate how we share our discoveries with colleagues, trainees, churches and communities. We reveal how our experiences and discoveries have developed the discernment process for chaplaincy vocation, urging the Church to see beyond the parish model in today's world. We reflect on chaplaincy in the pandemic in our context. We draw together our reflections on what we have learnt by telling our story and sustaining our willingness to learn.

"Creating space" means we use our context to tell our story and describe how our praxis evolves. By "creating space" daily as a forum for reflection, and here as a book, we model a practical theological reflection, showing that by telling our story and reflecting on our experiences, we reveal what we have learnt and how we develop our practice.

## Drawing together practice: the story so far

Over a year after joining the chaplaincy team, Sacha was asked to help with staff morale for a particular group of healthcare professionals, and so he instinctively offered reflective practice sessions. Developing a model of reflection for wellbeing and studying practical theology became the framework for his doctoral research. Creating knowledge through researching practice, as a chaplain reflecting with healthcare professionals, became an important milieu for the ongoing realization that every part of the chaplain's professional practice is a source of learning for the whole team. Practical theology and its paradigm in healthcare chaplaincy was a "coming home" to both authors.

In the very early days, the team opened the doors to parish clergy for the opportunity to refresh their experience of the pastoral care involved in hospital visiting, and invited them to consider practical theology and the "craft" (Bushell 2008) of the practice of chaplaincy. Soon after these early clergy study days, Jan joined the team.

The evolving department culture was already making gentle steps from a strong, faith-based ethos to one where the difference between pastoral, spiritual and religious care is clearly defined. The wider volunteer team, rather than coming almost exclusively from faith communities, began slowly to model a more diverse and inclusive representation.

Early in the reflective practice research, the daily debriefing of trained volunteers by a chaplain was slowly changing to become a place for the whole team as a reflective practice group. Here every pastoral encounter is a source of learning. Over these years, the pastoral training course similarly has moved from being strongly faith-influenced towards training with more visibly transferable skills. This means it is applicable for pastoral care in care homes, the hospital, the community, wherever listening skills and reflection are needed or indeed in any pastoral encounter regardless of context.

This evolving culture also involved a review of the chaplaincy's image and publicity, a careful exploration of the words used to describe the chaplaincy practice in context and a reduced focus on the individuals in post at any one time. It became clear that there was an increase in the transience of the chaplaincy community, not simply in the flow of patients welcoming support but also the staff and visitors. The team adopted the monastic hospitality model to describe the experience of people visiting the department, either to see a chaplain or use the chapel, or in some way be involved with the team for a while and then to leave at a time of their own choosing. This became known as the "wayfarer community".

The horizon broadened too with the team's contribution to regional chaplaincy conferences by using material from the pastoral care course to explore practice, looking more deeply into the pastoral encounter and the practitioner's development. Euphemistically referred to as Saltash to Buckfast (the venues over the years) these conferences started with limited success, not really appreciating what such a gathering could achieve. They have since become a valued opportunity to share in learning from discoveries.

Part of the evolution of nurturing pastoral visitors has been the introduction of volunteer mentoring, obviously prompted by volunteer legislation, but nevertheless with the desire to inspire a culture of learning together. As will be seen in later chapters, the basis of this is the reflective practice session for volunteers and chaplains at the end of the morning's ward visits. In this atmosphere of shared learning, each volunteer pastoral visitor is mentored, and everyone shares in the responsibility to learn and support each other. This is both in developing skills in practice, in the availability of study material and with the expectation of training and re-training. An example of this is in the smaller group, within the team, of end-of-life volunteers, in the belief that the more experienced pastoral visitor will grow to see their support of a dying patient, and family or visitors or staff, as an extension of their more day-to-day bedside visits. This is developing the same pastoral skills in the more acute or heightened awareness context, where both the apparently routine and the more sensitive scenarios inform each other and everyone's learning continues.

The relationship between members of the team, regardless of uniform or role, models the shared adventure for learning, whether an experienced volunteer or new chaplain. Everyone has the opportunity to identify their skills and develop in whatever way she or he is collaboratively discerned to be becoming.

Chaplaincy vocational discernment is a key feature of this adventure for learning for everyone in sharing the development of skills, but also in terms of both honorary and salaried healthcare chaplains. This is an important development for the Church, which has only just begun to see that the parish model is not the only paradigm of ministry. In later chapters, the experience of the growth of the pastoral visitor volunteer and the ordained minister into the gifted chaplain will be seen. This has been developed through newly ordained clergy being on placement with this team, the running of clergy study days and identifying the growing skills and passion for the work seen in the committed volunteer. Combining this has led to the creation of learning outcomes for chaplaincy discernment and professional development.

The story so far, drawing together practice, has outlined features of the early part of this ten-year adventure, indicating how this has informed changing practice through reflection and a desire to learn. In sharing these discoveries, these will be further demonstrated in later chapters. This introduction leads to the next reflection about the author practitioners; in other words, the chaplain's own story and how this informs their sense of healthcare chaplaincy in their own practical theology.

## The therapist and the reflective practitioner

The authors are both Anglican clergy who are passionate about healthcare chaplaincy and feel privileged to be called to be a priest in this context. They have healthcare backgrounds and are both naturally and professionally reflective. As chaplain practitioners, they share the ontological position that knowledge is gained by human experience with people exploring their own story and that of others. Here they want to combine this with the epistemology of sharing discoveries from the story of their work together. Building on the view that chaplaincy focusses too much on "doing" or proving its worth, rather than "being" (Stobert 2020: 77), the storytelling of these two practitioners aims to reveal a means of empowering the "being" of healthcare chaplaincy. These are their inner stories combined with the story of their work.

### Jan: psychology and psychotherapy to priest chaplain

Most clergy will attest to the notion that it is only with hindsight that the reality of a vocational journey seems to be more clearly evident and inherits some sort of shape, but that whilst at the beginning, or even in the middle, that picture is impossible to imagine. My story is no different.

I was a postdoctoral research fellow in a psychology department's Human Assessment Laboratory. We collaborated with international psychologists and enjoyed a reputation as an innovative research team. Despite our success, our Laboratory would in time be closed down in favour of other departmental foci, and team redundancy soon followed. But prior to knowing about our impending demise, I had been persuaded by several people that I had the temperament to train as a counsellor. I found work in a Community Mental Health Trust and was deployed to several GP surgeries to provide counselling to patients, as well as teaching counselling to students. Two years later, friends began encouraging me to consider ordination. Informal encouragement, whilst feeling initially like a set of unwelcome prods, began to feel both exciting and nerve-wracking. It was only when the exploration of ordination became more formal that this discernment journey became both challenging and painfully disheartening, rather than exciting.

From the beginning, clergy friends pointed out that any such ministry could fruitfully absorb and employ my psychology and counselling background. It would have been useful to have discussed this with someone in the ministry discernment process, and I had very much hoped to have this kind of initial exploratory conversation with the Diocesan Director of Ordinands (DDO). But during the first DDO meeting, I was offered no opportunity to explore whether ordained ministry could encompass an already existing counselling vocation; the interview focussed wholly on my perceived lack of certainty about being ordained, which was taken as evidence that I was not committed enough to explore my vocation! The norm from which the DDO worked was completely based on the parish model and so the idea of any kind of alternative ministry (parish alongside counselling or chaplaincy) remained unaddressed.

To inhabit the place where on the one hand, there is that inevitable quality of vocational discernment that feels like "this won't go away" and, on the other hand, the Church as an institution is telling you to "go away" because you're not sure enough about your vocation, is very distressing. It was only the kindness and intervention of clergy contacts that remedied this impasse. After more awkward meetings and a lukewarm reference from the DDO, I was finally granted an interview with the bishop, who sent me to a Bishop's Advisory Panel, and I was recommended for training.

Once ordained, I continued to be employed as a counsellor in the NHS alongside a self-supporting part-time parish curacy, but the part-time shape of parish work was not viewed favourably by the training incumbent, and it was a very unhappy time. I was given few opportunities to learn many of the skills needed for ordained ministry. My training incumbent told me that I should never have been ordained and therefore would not be recommending me for priesting—a decision that was overturned by the bishop.

I attended a curates' study day at the hospital, and in all kinds of unexpected and unasked for ways, it became clear that this needed to be explored further, so I volunteered as a hospital pastoral visitor. What followed was an increasing sense that this was the right place for me, and I was invited to transfer my curacy from the parish to the chaplaincy. *I want to emphasize that this transfer was not connected with experiencing a bad time in the parish.* I'm sure that there were failings on both sides, but if I explain that during my time in the parish, I was not allowed to conduct any funerals, baptisms, weddings or pastoral visits, it will be evident that the curacy was a very painful and disabling experience.

By contrast, the hospital chaplaincy welcomed me heartily and worked very hard to make sense of how a chaplaincy curacy might look. I was very much affirmed as curate by the department and offered some on-call work, which was a tremendous responsibility but one with which they trusted me. I shadowed chaplains and learnt how to do my first funeral, emergency baptism and end-of-life visiting. Just as important, I learnt a great deal through reflective practice, with which I was very much at home. I secured a part-time chaplaincy job in two psychiatric units, and my work life now combined being a psychiatric chaplain, an honorary chaplain in an acute hospital and an NHS counsellor in a number of GP surgeries. I was then encouraged to apply for and secured a full-time chaplaincy role in the hospital where I was completing my curacy.

Nine years later, I am utterly thankful that as a hospital chaplain, I am where I really believe I am best used. It has taken some time to recover the confidence lost in my parish curacy, but I have felt nothing but support and affirmation from my colleagues in applying my therapeutic and pastoral skills to this job and being willing to continue to learn. I feel that this work is often mistaken as a poor relation to parish-based ministry, and nothing could be further from the truth.

**Sacha: nursing and parish priest to priest chaplain researcher**
At ordination training selection, a senior selector said that his first thoughts of me were "nurse or priest or both". This followed my first career of sixteen years in critical care nursing and then a sense of being called to explore a vocational discernment to priesthood. This evolution would mean a life which, in my own words, "would take more of me, more of the time". During the latter years of nursing, I had felt that I was simply using the same skills and equipment each day, albeit taking care of different people in several contexts. However, I wanted to find a deeper sense of "me" within the whole of my daily life. I knew I could contribute to saving lives, but I had a thirst to know who these lives really were, each

as a human and unique person. Nursing had taught me many things, but perhaps most interestingly I had found the name for a thought process I had been following intuitively for most of my life. It is the personal insight and desire to explore self-awareness, to learn more from my own experiences, that is called reflective practice. It came naturally to me, and I wanted to help other people find that inner space and whatever this discovery might reveal for them.

After ten years in parish ministry, with all its celebrations and frustrations, and with an ongoing feel for working with others in vocational discernment, I also wanted to spend more time alongside those in need and to hear their story. This was another key crossroads on the journey. I had been encouraged to think I may have been suitable for a more senior clergy role but withdrew from a diocesan appointment halfway through the interview. I thought such a job would, to me, have been a move away from the coalface, working mostly only with clergy and people of faith! I felt called to something more agenda-free or congruent in the sense of being in the middle of people's real, earthy human lives. This means being where the centre is actually on the edge, like Malcolm Guite's Christmas poem describing the centre of the world being born on the edge of a small town and on the edge of human frailty and survival (Guite 2012: 15). This "place" is anywhere and everywhere, but it is the visceral interface of sacred and secular, at the very heart of human experience.

I think I have a very "incarnational" relationship with God, a sense of being accompanied in every corner of my life, and vocationally a deep desire to continue to evolve as the person God has called me to become. From chorister to priest, I have always loved church liturgy and music, and I see leading public worship in the same way, meaning accompanying others from the heart as we journey together. Just as the fifth-century church father Augustine of Hippo described the sacraments as "an outward sign of an inward grace", I feel continually moved at the phrase in the Eucharist, "We thank you for counting us worthy to stand in Your presence and serve You . . . " (Archbishops' Council 2000: 190). At the altar, I sense that I am some sort of channel, a thin space but with a human heart. I believe I continue to be called to empower others. I yearn for people to gain in confidence in telling their own story and to be open to finding the skills of reflective practice as a source of their discovery and learning.

Coming to work in a hospital again was not a step back but a vital step forward, because, as a priest, I feel called to be with those who, often unexpectedly, find they wish to be accompanied as they holistically discover something more of themselves. A recent encounter describes my interpretation today of the phrase "nurse or priest or both". I was contacted urgently by an experienced healthcare professional to support members of their team after a traumatic event in their department. Asked to be among them as they cleared away equipment and the bloody mess, I sat with them in the middle of their muddle. As they worked, they talked through what had happened, thinking through how they felt and on many levels considering what they were learning from their experiences, both in head and heart. Familiar with their critical care environment, my two professions came face to face. I knew I had been called to that moment but was also honoured to be there with that team on that day.

Practical theology, healthcare chaplaincy and research in reflective practice with healthcare professionals are among the joys and challenges of my ongoing, fulfilling and utterly privileged journey.

## What makes a chaplain?

"Listening to, interpreting and telling stories is the lifeblood of chaplaincy" (Swinton 2015: 300).

"We improve our effectiveness as practitioners of the arts of ministry by taking time to reflect upon our practice" (Sullender 2017: 105).

If human life finds credibility and connection by the stories of human experiences (Bochner and Riggs 2014; Swinton 2015) and if the chaplain's professional life is involved with those stories, then they are contextually at the very heart of human experience. Chaplains are "skilled boundary crossers" whose work is "messy . . . impure and fascinating" (Pattison 2015b: 116). We write here our story, our experiences, our shared learning, but before exploring our sense of what makes a chaplain, we place our story alongside the current focus of healthcare chaplaincy.

## The focus of healthcare chaplaincy

Broadly the themes, perhaps inevitably, focus on issues that identify the role amidst challenges to the profession's value. These include provision of spiritual care of the patient, apologetics for chaplaincy in the secular institution, and chaplaincy training and self-development through supervision (Kelly 2012; Kelly and Paterson 2013; Paterson 2015). Other themes include working with critical care and the vulnerable such as paediatrics, in end-of-life care and mental health, and the development of relationships in spiritual care and multifaith issues in healthcare, demonstrating contextual and holistic "care for all" (Fitchett and Nolan 2015; Pye, Sedgewick and Todd 2015). Chaplains' support of staff is a key part of the role but its increasingly vital place should not be underestimated, "helping them process difficult situations and emotions from personal and professional experiences" (McClung, Grossoehme and Jacobson 2006: 151). The way in which Sacha's doctoral research contributed to developing reflective practice to nurture healthcare professionals' wellbeing, and thus chaplains' support of staff, will be described in a later chapter.

A nursing review outlines key areas of the healthcare chaplain's role internationally describing it as pastoral and religious care, work in the multifaith context and with some uncertainty in relation to how well chaplains support nurse spiritual care training (Timmins et al. 2017). The authors see chaplains as providing care and support where people are often in life-changing circumstances and conclude that the chaplain's role will prove important because of an increase of ethical issues where chaplains are alongside everyone involved both clinically and personally. They advocate chaplaincy research that connects with the care of the whole person.

Chaplaincy has been defined as "care involving the intentional recognition and articulation of the sacred by nominated individuals authorized for the task in secular situations" (Cobb, Swift and Todd 2015: 2). It is in a place where faith is not the main agenda and yet where faith is diversely available (Gilliat-Ray and Arshad 2015: 109). This connects with the public accessibility and openness of the chaplain, who is frequently approached in the hospital by those who would never usually seek contact with the Church. Chaplaincy is an example of public theology, the interface between religion and the public space, the hospital as a new forum for these encounters described as "chaplaincy in the public square" (Todd 2011).

Here theology is a way of thinking, where for chaplains "theology is their expertise" and as "a source of nurture, challenge and insight" (Pattison 2015b: 111, 126) with religion as an example and not an end in itself. This links with the sense of the Church as being a resource rather than expecting faithful response (Billings 2004: 113). This does not deny the integrity of the faith of the chaplain but invites the insights of faith to provide the language of transformation and change, journeying and discovery. It is a source of new life revealed in the public place. Chaplaincy is the care of the whole person, with "a focus on the ultimate value of the person" rather than how they connect with any other structure or teaching (Pattison 2015a: 26). The chaplain is not in the business of active evangelism. Their work is by their presence "standing alongside individuals and institutions to nurture citizenship and human flourishing", to "seek and promote justice for the disenfranchised" with "enacted parables of care and witness" as their "creative endeavour" (Pattison 2015b: 126).

The chaplain has also been described as "healer" in this ministry, identifying health as the presence of wellbeing "even in the midst of illness" (Swinton and Kelly 2015: 183, 181). This is an invitation to the whole of healthcare with the chaplain as a "cultural broker . . . who facilitates the crossing of boundaries" between different people or "between different understandings of health . . . different perspectives on the nature of healing, recovery and wellbeing . . ." (Swinton and Kelly 2015: 183). The chaplain is then also "educator, resource and support of staff . . . with the . . . skills to equip other staff to fruitfully inhabit such a health world, deliver person-centred, holistic, spiritual care . . ." (Swinton and Kelly 2015: 183, 184). Finding health as wellbeing "even in the midst of extreme difficulties" (Swinton and Kelly 2015: 184) is a significant role for the chaplain. Sacha's reflective practice research identified the wider understanding of wellbeing to also be holistic, relational and contextual, allowing for building space in which healthcare professionals can move towards nurturing wellbeing within themselves (Pearce 2018).

In gathering stories of chaplaincy practice, in the face of the changes and challenges of the twenty-first century, there is a call for chaplaincy development in terms of "working as spiritual agents of transformation" in order to "promote individual and collective wellbeing" (Kelly and Swinton 2020: 25). They promote an emphasis on a chaplaincy image of doing "soul work" meaning that "true health and wellbeing can only be found through a holistic approach", with chaplains as central to this (Kelly and Swinton 2020: 26, 27).

*Creating Space* is just this sort of chaplaincy story, sharing discoveries about empowering others, learning through reflection and self-discovery. With the chaplain as a reflective companion, it is a unique model of ministry and a personal, human one.

## The unique model of ministry

From the start of his healthcare chaplaincy ministry in 2009, Sacha saw the chaplain as having a unique model of ministry—a very particular presence, in an uncertain and changing place, of a particular kind of person. Creating a personal model, he built on the priest model that had been developed as "witness, watchman and weaver" (Lewis-Anthony 2009: 83). These became his chaplain images of "explorer, archaeologist and safari guide". The explorer is a lookout and map reader, helping to see the way. The archaeologist is an interpreter who gently holds, brushing dust away to help see the broken pieces and helping identify the treasure. The safari guide journeys alongside, helping to see, identify and discover. This is a guide in the wilderness who helps make connections with what was seen yesterday and today. In a different way, evolving a model within his research project, he became more able to articulate a deeper awareness of the personal element of the "human vulnerable chaplain" in his relationship with healthcare professionals.

A ministry of "being there" (Speck 1988) has long described chaplaincy as a particular "ministry of presence" and as a "non-anxious presence" (Newell cited in Mowat, Bunniss, Snowden and Wright 2013), that "meets people where they are" (Mowat and Swinton 2007: 30). It is a "craft", where the chaplain develops a "quality of presence", so it is a reflexive ministry

(Bushell 2008: 60). It is a watching, listening presence where spiritual care could be called "a way of naming absences and recognizing gaps" (Swinton and Pattison 2010: 226). They add "We might use the image of putting a rope around an area of deserted land in order to allow wildlife to develop and flourish" (Swinton and Pattison 2010: 234). It means "being present while the other person works it out for him or herself" (Orchard cited in Swift 2009: 175). For the "primary skills of the chaplain [are] presence, listening, empathy, spiritual discernment" (Swinton 2015: 300).

This is a "wilderness ministry" that needs "watchfulness" by "those who stand on the margins who see the wider picture" (Moody 1999: 15, 22) in this "insecure and uncertain landscape" (Swift 2009: 122). It is someone capable of working with a "sense of homelessness, the constant crossing and re-crossing of boundaries, the need for hospitality, the importance of chance encounters" (Moody 1999: 23). It is someone "who know[s] what it means to inhabit uncertainty and change" (Swift 2009: 169). It is a ministry that may constantly "walk through ordinary doors to spend time in rooms with those whose lives have suddenly become immersed in sorrow" (Swift 2009: 169). This is a ministry as "chaplain standing in the world ... and looking around" (Walters 2017: 51).

The chaplain is especially skilled in the gathering and welcome nature of the pastoral encounter, in creating that space, and naming the reality. This means developing skills in helping people in crisis tell their story: "Speaking in signs, communicating in the language of silence, preserving the gestures of pain ... attempts to let suffering speak" (Walton, H. 2002: 4). It is a person able to work with dialogue that may not involve words, as well as someone who can deal with what is hard to hear, tough conversations and difficult encounters.

The chaplain is a companion on the way, able to facilitate the discovery that, through one's own reflections, one may be able to interpret experiences and develop wellbeing in the face of acute challenge, to "give sacramental recognition to moments of personal crisis" (Swift 2009: 167). This means using the skills of one able to notice change and transformation of any kind. This is a person who is sufficiently able to deal with their own story in order to be able to hear the story of others.

## The reflective companion

The chaplain is a reflective practitioner by the very nature of their own vocational discernment and profession. They have a background in theological reflection, which is an essential practice for the developing deep connection between human experience and a relationship with God. This is reflection as a "discipline" which is "a deliberate process of critically interpreting and understanding experience" (Cobb 2005: 29). Here reflection is fundamental to daily professional practice, vocational discernment, self-awareness and wellbeing. As someone who practises critical thinking, and is familiar with reflecting for professional and personal development, the chaplain is a resource for nurturing this in others.

For chaplains, reflective practice has been described as a "core skill" using "case studies" for professional development (Slater 2015: 66; Swift 2015: 170). It is also part of professional validity in best practice, determining "how to respond to the unique circumstances of certain individuals in particular places and specific situations" (Cobb, Swift and Todd 2015: 1). Reflection is understood as a tool for chaplaincy "supervision" as means of essential support (Paterson 2015: 153). It is described as a tool for chaplains' own development. However, more recently reflection has been defined as "a developing state of mind", which combines reflection in and on action with critical thinking and reflexivity (Stobert 2020: 63). Such a model draws together both the active and post-event reflection with further subsequent "review of events and pastoral exchanges" (Stobert 2020: 65) and the deeper processes of self-knowing and change.

The chaplain as a reflective companion also offers the personal human connection by being approachable and realistic, genuine in their own openness and presence. Here also the chaplain is "empty handed" (Swift 2009: 175) and the "welcoming guest" of "mutual hospitality" (Walton, M. 2012: 226). These particular images are significant in the *Creating Space* story and feature elsewhere in later chapters, including in Chapter 5, which discusses our pastoral care training. Having outlined the key role and qualities of the chaplain as far as we discern, we now focus on these two motifs of "empty hands" and "hospitality" to consider how they contribute to our "creating space" image and are vital to our practice.

## Creating Space: empty hands

During the COVID-19 pandemic, "space" is a subject of both importance and challenge, whether related to the two-metre space required between people for physical social distancing or the space of empty days yawning ahead for people at home, isolated. Finding space has been a matter of human interest in differing ways before, such as space for the "health tourism" of spa, retreat or relaxation technique (Smith and Puczko) or else exploring life beyond earth's frontiers for sci-fi enthusiasts. The thesis title from Sacha's reflective practice research includes the phrase "building space", because he was developing a reflective model as a chaplain who empowers others to find space and to nurture their wellbeing. Emerging from the literature early in his research were the motifs of chaplain as "empty handed" (Swift 2009: 175) and the "welcoming guest" of "mutual hospitality" (Walton, M. 2012: 226) which he combined, developing the sense of the "pastoral encounter" as a relational and hospitality ministry.

These images model the chaplain who celebrates the richness of humanity in the other person, willing to give time and space to hear their story. This is especially so when that story is challenging because where "there are no answers, no quick exits to open, [this] does not require the gifts of those whose hands are full" (Swift 2009: 175). Instead, it "calls for great patience, compassion and faithfulness to the value of the human being" from the chaplain, which is a "product of considerable preparation, maturity and deep personal self-knowledge" (Swift 2009: 175). It is someone skilled in creating space into which others tell their story and feel accompanied in their storytelling as they develop their own reflective self-care skills: "For only when the chaplain's hands are empty will wounded people dare to offer their stories and allow their most intimate shards of doubt and hope to be handled with love and honoured with insight" (Swift 2009: 175).

Developing the "empty hands" model, as we have reflected and fostered in our practice, means creating space before, during and after the pastoral encounter. Taking time with reflective self-preparation, even if only briefly, before listening to someone in a pastoral encounter, can create space within oneself, within one's own sense of self-awareness. This means being sufficiently able to put aside one's own story, making space to listen to the other person, becoming the "empty hands" for them to fill with their story. The listener holds the broken treasure of someone's story in their hands while the teller finds the tools in order to be able to hold it themselves. As Swift (2009) implies, if one is burdened with one's own issues, one cannot give honour and full attention to the other, unable to listen properly, with insufficient emotional intelligence not to be overwhelmed by the challenge of what is being said. A chaplain who may have something even slightly onerous on their mind cannot give space to hold someone else's story.

This is further drawn out in the "welcoming guest" model, where both the chaplain and the other person in the pastoral encounter share "mutual hospitality" (Walton, M. 2012: 226).

## Creating Space: mutual hospitality

The chaplain is "an interested guest, as a stranger in a strange land" but who equally is able "to welcome the stranger ... to host the strange" (Walton, M. 2012: 228, 233). Taking a gentle approach to any pastoral encounter, the listening chaplain carefully enters the other person's space, drawing alongside them as guest, but is also the host by beginning to create the space for the other person to feel able to tell their story. This connects with offering unconditional welcome and inclusion, meeting without judgement, and with the chaplain's willingness to be turned away because the hospitality is on the other person's terms. This means also the chaplain has the responsibility to be sensitive, even tentative towards creating the space.

Creating this space *within* the pastoral encounter involves being the "non-anxious presence" (Newell cited in Mowat et al. 2013: 39), that "meets people where they are" (Mowat and Swinton 2007: 30). It means listening to the other person tell their story as, and if, they feel desirous to do so. Listening includes allowing space for silences and sometimes encouraging the speaker with gentle prompting, for example by carefully asking why perhaps the issue has been raised or is on their mind today. It is the other person's agenda and at their pace, with the listener "being present while the other person works it out for him or herself" (Orchard cited in Swift 2009: 175). This is where it is "far more important that a person discovers what he needs rather than be given someone else's answers which may turn out to be a bad fit" (Long 1990: 34).

Focussed listening with occasional gentle prompting, inviting the other person to tell their story if they desire, helping the storyteller "hear" what they have said, allowing space for silence, all involves reflection-in-action within the pastoral encounter. It means considering what is being said and not being said, seeing connections, and reflecting where, how, and whether to prompt. To go beyond this would potentially be to refill the "empty hands" of the listener. Giving advice, opinions or solutions turns the encounter to the listener's agenda and not the storyteller's, refilling the hands and turning attention away from the speaker. Having the "empty hands" to be filled with the other's story means that the hands can only hold and show, not point or direct.

By combining in practice these two models of "empty handed" (Swift 2009: 175), and "welcoming guest" (Walton, M. 2012: 226), the chaplain can create the space in the pastoral encounter. However, this challenges the view that the space merely occurs, for example in Whorton's view of himself: "I do not create this space. If I try to manufacture it, nothing will be created. It is a place that I glimpse out of the corner of my eye" (Whorton 2011: 38). Equally, such a space has been seen as indicative of the chaplain's "vacuum identity" where they "fill a void rather than offering a well-defined service" (de Vries, Berlinger and Cadge 2008: 25). Yet we *do* create this space, the "non-anxious presence" (Newell cited in Mowat et al. 2013: 39), listening, shaping the response, reflecting and making connections, being the "empty hands" that hold and show rather than point. Such a claim is supported by those who see "space" as being created by listening:

> The essence of what chaplains offer—generic spiritual listening—can be described as active non-judgemental listening that creates a 'dynamic holding space' which ... the storyteller, can use to talk about the present and to revisit and reinterpret events from the past, and in so doing maintain their story or create new possibilities, even a new sense of hope, for the future (Kennedy and Stirling 2013: 62, 63).

This is a vital space where wellbeing may be nurtured: "Understanding the link between wellbeing and the act of listening gives theoretical substance to the core work of chaplaincy" (Mowat et al. 2013: 35). This is a place of nurture, with "spirituality as a way of naming absences and recognizing gaps in healthcare" with "the image of putting a rope around an area of deserted land in order to allow wildlife to develop and flourish" (Swinton and Pattison 2010: 226, 234). This is a space for discovery, development and change. It is also a "blurred encounter" (Reader and Baker 2009). As such it is the "Third Space . . . the space that exists in the middle of any set of binary opposites", a space which "is constantly evolving and changing" (Reader and Baker 2009: 4, 5). These are "blurred encounters to thresholds of transformation" (Reader and Baker 2009: 219). Here, the

> threshold represents the space of new insight and opportunity from which to engage in transforming and purposive action . . . never the end of the journey . . . the start of another journey into a new set of encounters (Reader and Baker 2009: 220).

For the chaplain, then, the reflective "created space" is also an example of "a new theological space" (Reader and Baker 2009) that has been identified in twenty-first century social and public theology, sharing the interface of mixed perspectives and finding a place for mutual learning. It is a place of hospitality and space for change.

As a chaplain, as one "who know[s] what it means to inhabit uncertainty and change" (Swift 2009: 169), this is a person whose own journey and profession involves a relational ministry. It is one who is alongside and who identifies transformation. Sharing the opportunity for learning and change, this invites the possibility of developing oneself and others in the reflective space. This connects with the listening nature of chaplaincy, as in any context "being listened to and telling our story is in itself therapeutic and life affirming" (Mowat et al. 2013: 35), where the listener holds the story, allowing the teller to make their discoveries. Moreover, "Listening is a foot washing ministry . . . to do with attitudes . . . availability, compassion, belief in people—knowing from our own experience what being heard can do for us" (Long 1990: 35). Here, the priority is given to the other, but if this were to be mutual, surely both would be heard and loved. However, listening has been described in terms of "gift, hospitality and healing" (Long 1990: 35). This is "mutual rather than one-way, for the listener in giving also receives—the trust, confidence and vulnerability of the one who turns to him" (Long 1990: 36). A chaplain will know this sense of privilege of being told someone's story and therefore "gifted" with material for one's own reflections and learning. It is a shared place of hospitality and change. Creating space *after* the pastoral encounter involves reflection-on-action, making each encounter a source of learning.

## Creating Space: hospitality and change

Hospitality, as a term first recognized in the fourteenth century (Merriam-Webster Dictionary 2017) describing feeding and housing people journeying on the road, is the source from which hospital and hospice originate. The philosopher Jacques Derrida declares "an act of hospitality can only be poetic" (Derrida and Dufourmantelle 2000: 2), describing this complex meeting place of strangers. He states:

> absolute hospitality requires that I open up my home and that I give not only to the foreigner ... but to the absolute, unknown, anonymous other ... and that I *give place* to them, that I let them come, that I let them arrive, and take place in the place I offer them, without asking of them either reciprocity ... or even their names (Derrida and Dufourmantelle 2000: 25).

Derrida sees hospitality as a paradox because it makes the host the unwelcome stranger. This connects with reflections on "mutual hospitality" (Walton, M. 2012: 226) where, in the pastoral encounter and the reflective space, the chaplain paradoxically both fills the gaps and creates the space in that tentative step as both host and guest.

As part of his own inner life and journeying, the Dutch theologian and priest Henri Nouwen saw creating space as making room for others, sharing humanity, offering the possibility for both to be changed. Moving from "hostility into hospitality" (Nouwen 1998: 43), both "guest and host can reveal their most precious gifts and bring new life to each other" (Nouwen 1998: 45). This is "a fundamental attitude towards our fellow human beings" (Nouwen 1998: 45). This meeting or encounter, this hospitality, is "the creation of a free space where the stranger can enter and become a friend . . . Hospitality is not to change people, but to offer them space where change can take place" (Nouwen 1998: 49). This is a place of "mutual hospitality" (Walton, M. 2012: 226) and the potential of mutual learning. This is "friendly emptiness where strangers can enter and discover themselves as created free . . . free also to leave and follow their own vocations" (Nouwen 1998: 49).

Creating space means letting go of the busy life, letting go of the fear of space (Nouwen 1998: 50), if only briefly, and, like being "empty handed" (Swift 2009: 175), means there is room for something new to be discovered. In their context, of teaching in adult learning, Groen and Kawalilak (2016) consider how giving room for one another, and hearing one another's story, can be a place of real transformation and self-learning by "intentionally slowing down the pace", offering room for discovery (Groen and Kawalilak 2016: 62).

In the pastoral encounter or reflecting with staff or colleagues, the chaplain "slows down the pace" in a sense, making space for discovery. Reflecting on the "profound intimacy" of the space between nurse and patient, Swinton and Vanderpot observe:

> It is the space between that matters. The space between is the place of meeting; it is a space that is not created by distance, but by a mutual movement towards one another in an attempt to create space for care that values, respects, and offers hospitality towards both participants (Swinton and Vanderpot 2017: 215).

It is that very space, within those professional relationships, in which the chaplain also is present, honouring that working "space" and offering those involved the opportunity to build from it. It is possible to develop another space where reflection on the earlier experience provides exploration and discovery, with the new space as a source for learning. This builds on the idea of an encounter being an offer of hospitality to one another for mutual discovery and change. Perhaps this is a messy place, but it is human. It is a space where all are welcome, each story is valid and valued, the richness of shared humanity is celebrated, and there is a willingness to be changed by the experience. This becomes a reflective space, creating a hospitable, transformation place where an encounter is a source of learning.

## Creating Space: reflective space and the pastoral encounter as a source of learning

The word "encounter" originates from terms to describe meeting in conflict, the unexpected and the adversarial (Merriam-Webster Dictionary 2017). Contextually, as a chaplain, the "chance encounter" is the unexpected engagement with a patient, a visitor or member of staff. Any encounter can be described as a pastoral encounter because the work of the chaplain is a "ministry of care" (Cobb 2005: 42). From September 2016, following Sacha's research, we suggested calling our department's training volunteer course "Creating Space: The Pastoral Encounter" in order to describe the sense of the pastoral encounter as a space and a source for learning through reflection. Our images of the listener being a "vomit bowl" or "garbage bins" (Department of Pastoral and Spiritual Care 2016) are perhaps less attractive, yet they come from significant reflections on pastoral encounters from within our team. These images describe the holding of something that needs to be expressed, got out, removed and looked over. They indicate something of the processing, the space that is "reflective practice", and also a sense of liberation in the storyteller.

In chaplaincy, regardless of the context, the listening presence *is* the pastoral encounter, with the pastoral care as the focussed listening, and spiritual care as this space to help the storyteller to listen to themselves. The reflective space is precisely that listening space, for discovery, shared learning and nourishment. This is our professional practice, to listen to others and help them listen to themselves, and our motivation to empower others to discover this for themselves.

The reflective space that is a pastoral encounter with chaplain and healthcare professionals or colleagues combines practical theology's roots in theological reflection and healthcare's foundation of reflective practice as a method of education. It returns reflection to deeply embrace the "experience" that Dewey (1933, 1938) advocated and the "reflection-in-action" that Schön (1983) saw as the source of knowledge. It returns reflection to the "story of the heart" that is key to theological reflection (Graham, Walton and Ward 2005). These images will be returned to in the concluding chapter.

Through research in healthcare, we have grown to see more widely the pastoral encounter as a source of learning through reflective practice. The value of the chaplain reflecting on their own pastoral practice is familiar in their professional development (Kelly 2010; Kelly and Paterson 2013). The pastoral encounter is a tool for learning because "pastoral practice not reflected upon is practice that only partially fulfils its potential" (Kelly 2010: 48). Developing reflection, based on using Sacha's HELP model (see Chapter 3), in our chaplaincy practice of reflection in the team of chaplains and pastoral visitors, we have seen how the pastoral encounter is repeatedly the source of ongoing learning in this mixed group. Creating space and growing skills in the reflective group, who daily develop their practice through reflection, enables them to consider how today will make them a better pastoral carer tomorrow. Each of today's pastoral encounters informs and develops practice for tomorrow. The reflective space develops the relationship between those involved, not simply with self as a functional tool but self as relational and organic, in caring for one another, caring for ourselves and sharing in developing transferable skills.

## Creating Space: the human chaplain

The congruent, genuine, organic chaplain develops professional relationships by creating space. Building relational trust, they identify the space and create it by a presence of accessibility, openness and hospitality, for the storyteller to share stories and experiences, recognizing and identifying the richness of our shared humanity. The chaplain is carer for that space, the one who creates it and notices its presence—and the one who identifies transformation there. They are the "welcoming guest", sharing the space, and arrive there relationally and by showing vulnerability and humanity. A pastoral encounter is never about "my" story; rather it is hearing and welcoming the storyteller and their story. Whether in any pastoral encounter, or else reflecting with staff or colleagues, the chaplain creates the hospitable space where any story can be told.

Thus far, with this understanding of healthcare chaplaincy, we have highlighted the way in which our department has evolved over the last ten years, and these themes will be developed in further chapters. We have placed this introductory outline alongside the personal vignettes of the authors' journeys into and commitment to healthcare chaplaincy. From there we have described the essential characteristics of the chaplain who has a heartfelt willingness to join the adventure for learning, every step of the way, through the unfolding of their story in reflection and in context with the desire to evolve practice, for stories to be told and practice to evolve.

We now offer ideas and suggestions on the way in which our "Creating Space" material may be used. We shall then connect this, our evolving practice, with an understanding of practical theology.

## How to use this book and share discoveries

"Creating Space" is a story that shares our discoveries and wants to make them accessible to others. We are "creating space" for those in any form of caring work or ministry to consider our practice of chaplaincy as a model to explore in their own context. Not least of which, *Creating Space: Story, Reflection and Practice in Healthcare Chaplaincy* is a message to the Church, opening our door inviting the institution to see chaplaincy as a model of ministry for this century, living the Gospel, developing pastoral care for all. We outline each section here and suggest ways in which our discoveries could be developed.

- Chapter 1 includes our understanding of the unique role of the healthcare chaplain and ways in which we continue to develop this with our model of "creating space".

- Chapter 2 sets out in a straightforward way our view of healthcare chaplaincy as a model of practical theology, highlighting the connection between the two.
- Chapter 3 describes the motivation and methodology of a chaplain's research project in reflective practice in healthcare in a way that means it could be reproduced elsewhere.
- Chapter 4 identifies what "being" means to us, sharing our definitions of pastoral and spiritual care, our use of reflective practice, our nurture of volunteers, how we learn together and our wayfarer image of our community.
- Chapter 5 summarizes our pastoral care training course, which consists of six two-hour sessions.
- Chapter 6 sets out three regional chaplaincy conferences (for chaplains and volunteer pastoral visitors) that we have facilitated.
- Chapter 7 describes the discoveries we made as we shared our learning with parishes and dioceses, and the way in which we learnt more about how to learn together.
- Chapter 8 explores the journey of discovery in discerning the "chaplain"; looks at our experiences of curates on placement; shares our insights with other clergy; recounts the journey of a gifted volunteer pastoral visitor discerning her vocation, and looks at our process of developing learning outcomes for the discernment and curacy of a chaplain. This chapter is a plea to help the Church identify another model of ministry beyond the parish.
- Chapter 9 shares reflections and discoveries in our context of living and working with COVID-19 as chaplains.
- Chapter 10 reflects on what we have learnt by telling our story and suggesting future work and research.

CHAPTER 2

# Defining practical theology

## The contextual dialogue of narrative and praxis (Graham 2005, 2012)

Healthcare chaplaincy is a rich paradigm of practical theology in the changing and challenging hinterland of acute human experience. Drawing from his reflective practice research, under the canopy of practical theology, Sacha has found this definition illuminating as it mirrors the work of the healthcare chaplain:

> Practical theology has "always been contextual" (Graham et al. 2005: 10), "studying lived experience" while " ... holding the immediacy of praxis and narrative in creative tension ... " (Graham 2012: 198).

This amalgam of Elaine Graham's own developing work shows how this understanding of theology is itself an immense resource and example of the adventure of learning, "in ministry or action" within "the human context and the realities of lived experience" (Graham 2017: 173). At its heart, practical theology's tool is theological reflection for "induction and nurture", "building and sustaining" and "communicating" (Graham et al. 2005: 10) and is for both the individual and communities. Healthcare chaplains, who reflect and learn together from every pastoral encounter, are examples of precisely this resource for learning and developing practice. This is learning through human experience and explores the human story.

Taking illustrations from practical theologians Elaine Graham, Richard Osmer and Eric Stoddart shows human experience as a tool for transformation by engaging with the human story for each in the pastoral encounter.

## Listening, learning, leading: the core tasks (Osmer 2008)

From his own practical theology, Rick Osmer (2008) developed a model of learning through the realities and complexities of the pastoral encounter. He uses vivid human stories, reflecting on real pastoral encounters, as tools for learning for the development of clergy as better pastoral care providers. He advocates his "core tasks" of being alongside others with "careful listening" (Osmer 2008: 73), interpreting through "thoughtfulness" and "wise judgement" (Osmer 2008: 82–5), and through "cross-disciplinary dialogue" (Osmer 2008: 172). The final "task" is leading by the visibility of one's own humanity and vulnerability towards "an ability to empower others" (Osmer 2008: 192). From listening and reflection comes learning at deepening levels and an ongoing willingness to discover. This holds together human experience and reflection, while being alongside others in the process of growth and change. This is central to the work of the healthcare chaplain in listening and empowering others.

Osmer's own journey is through Gerkin's hermeneutical relation between pastor and people with priest as "interpretive guide" (Osmer 2008: 33). He develops the connectedness of Miller-McLemore's "living human web" onto his wider term, "web of life" (Osmer 2008: 33). This means being alert to the reality and complexities surrounding the layers of the pastoral encounter. He asks clergy to respond to this "challenge of double reflexivity" (Osmer 2008: 240), which means seeing the change in oneself and in one's community. Developing this in the healthcare context, Sacha's research explored the priest/chaplain who, through the pastoral encounter of the reflective space with healthcare professionals, moves towards a form of reflective practice that fosters a new sense of wellbeing. This is a "double reflexivity" for both in the pastoral encounter, creating space, sharing and reflecting on human stories, and finding change in themselves and in their work community. By both professions developing their own practice, they are sources of mutual learning in their reflective pastoral encounter.

## Living human documents (Boisen; Graham)

This relates to Elaine Graham's further development of the phrase "living human document", which she takes beyond the clergy study model, describing it "as an entry-point into a deeper apprehension of the very meaning of human existence" (Graham 2009: 151). Further, it is "any instance of pastoral practice or encounter, regardless of its actual agent or locus" (Graham 2009: 151), therefore a source of learning in any context. Valued in whatever way they are presented, "those 'texts' are always embodied, gendered and contextual" (Graham 2009: 151). This is discovery through human experience, in whatever way it may be identified and interpreted, so anyone can become their own learning resource.

Returning the "living human document" to its origins in chaplaincy and healthcare re-associates with Anton Boisen's intentions. The twentieth-century chaplain and educator saw this "document" as a personal and professional source of learning. Using his own story, finding the medical treatment of his mental ill health "cold, clinical and lacking in meaning" he felt "called to consider who he had become" with so much more to be gained by "deep self-scrutiny" (O'Laughlin 2005: 48, 49). He explored his life and studies, the people around him and his own self-awareness, and in his reflections found that "understanding his own life, in all its detailed singularity, had been the key to his recovery" (O'Laughlin 2005: 49). Developing the value of the individual story, both personal and in case study, he saw the "living human document" as an essential learning resource (O'Laughlin 2005: 49, 50).

Healthcare chaplains, as practical theologians, empower people to recognize the human story as a source of learning and this discovery as a shared experience. Regardless of faith or institution, people sharing this together are on "pilgrimage: journeying, on the move, telling and sharing stories and occasionally visiting sacred places" (Graham 2009: 152). Graham develops this as "inclusive and non-sectarian" but nevertheless "with all those who identify themselves as the people of God" (Graham 2009: 152). However, it can be argued that this is possible for those journeying together where not everyone would identify themselves as people of faith (Pearce 2018: 24). The shared experience of chaplain as the reflective companion in the pastoral encounter, with whomever, could be described, as has been said of God's Kingdom, as "living at the threshold between sacred and secular" (Graham 2011: 233). Further, at such an interface any contribution from the faith perspective "must be offered in the name of a common humanity and shared concern for its flourishing" (Graham 2011: 233). If at that interface, then, the chaplain is the practitioner engaged in that "shared concern".

## Listening and hospitality

From his own story, Eric Stoddart (2014) shares insights into his transformation and flourishing, and its effect on his faith background (Stoddart 2014: 12). He describes learning "the power of reflective listening", moving his understanding in the pastoral encounter from giving advice to the "hospitality of listening" and "creating space for another" (Stoddart 2014: 5). For him, it was "a shift from listening for God to being silent for God", seeing his own ecclesiology and theology move to "creating space wherein a person could come to insight" (Stoddart 2014: 6). Stoddart is the listener in the pastoral encounter who is deeply changed by the experience. He moves in his understanding and experience of the pastoral encounter and pastoral care. This mirrors Osmer's "challenge of double reflexivity" (Osmer 2008: 240) for both in the pastoral encounter, as well as Graham's "embodied, gendered and contextual" nature of "living human documents" (Graham 2009: 151). It links also with the "mutual hospitality" (Walton, M. 2012: 226) and the "embrace" of the pastoral encounter as "a time for understanding and communion", the work of the chaplain being through their "subtle hospitality of ... presence" (Whipp 2017: 116). Once again, we see that each encounter is a unique source of learning.

## Practical theology: always willing to learn

With healthcare chaplaincy as a model of practical theology, with the continued desire to learn through the contextual dialogue of narrative and praxis (Graham et al. 2005; Graham 2012), the *Creating Space* story is an example of always being willing to learn. This continuously has reflection at its heart. It exemplifies the relationship between practical theology and reflective practice which creates "knowledge that is useful for people in the conduct of their lives and to enhance their holistic wellbeing in community" (Stobert 2020: 75). Our *Creating Space* story reflects on ten years of the healthcare chaplaincy practice of two chaplains, their wider department and shared context, identifying what they have learnt and how their praxis has evolved. We share the story of our experiences and our reflections, showing how this has developed our daily practice. Through this we also demonstrate that we are always willing to learn, believing that our practical theology is our daily practice, reflecting and learning at the heart of human experience in the context of the hospital community. Opening our door, we invite pastoral caregivers in any context, including the Church community, to see our story, our reflections and developing practice as a practical theology for their context too. We encourage the Church of today to avoid being, at best, simply buildings for its faithful membership and, at worst, "a dispenser of religious goodies" (Speck 1988: 31) but rather to develop its practice as chaplain to everyone. After all, to love my neighbour (Luke 10:27) does not mean to persuade them to believe what we may believe, not to be insistent "peddlers of truth", but rather to "create space" for the pastoral encounter to be an exciting, rewarding source of hospitality and discovery.

Thus far, we have offered an accessible understanding of practical theology as a willingness to learn and develop practice through human experience. This has been demonstrated with examples from practical theologians who engage with the human story of the pastoral encounter. We have placed ourselves in our own context, identifying how our story reveals this capacity for reflection and constant learning. We will now offer in further detail the story of our own reflective practice model as a tool for our learning.

CHAPTER 3

# Reflective practice: chaplain research in healthcare

It is a combination of practitioners' work, chaplaincy studies and the call for further research that encourages the exploration of the place of religious professionals working in a secular context where, as we identified in Chapter 1, faith is not the main agenda and yet where faith is diversely available (Gilliat-Ray and Arshad 2015: 109). The place of the chaplain at the interface of secular and sacred has also been identified, with chaplains as a resource for holistic care in the public space (for example Billings 2004; Todd 2011; Pattison 2015b) who are also able to identify the sacred, whatever that may mean to anyone, while not directly pointing to issues of faith (Todd, Cobb and Swift 2015: 333). This has been the experience within this story of *Creating Space* with chaplain research in healthcare. Both authors, Sacha and Jan, from their respective backgrounds, brought their experience of using reflective practice to the team. What became the next step for the department was Sacha's research as chaplain developing this with healthcare professionals, which took the form of his doctoral research question, "Building Space: Developing Reflection for Wellbeing. Can a chaplain help healthcare professionals develop reflective practice for wellbeing for themselves and their team?" (Pearce 2018). He developed a process of reflective practice for staff, arguing for a broader interpretation of wellbeing that was more holistic, relational and contextual. This also developed reflective practice beyond its use in healthcare for education and professional development. Researching with teams of healthcare professionals, he developed the simple and memorable HELP Wellbeing Reflection Cycle and identified the value of creating provision for reflective space to nurture wellbeing in the care, and self-care, of healthcare staff. In this chapter, he tells this story, offering his reflections and the way this practice has developed. The methodology is offered in detail in order that it may be reproduced and developed in other contexts.

## Staff wellbeing: research motivation

In my professional context as a hospital chaplain, I seemed to be breaking new ground in using reflective practice as a tool endeavouring to raise the morale of healthcare professionals. I was also developing its practice with pastoral visitor volunteers. My motivations came in early 2010 from two distinct events. At a local chaplaincy conference, I was observed by Dr Harriet Mowat, who, seeing me encouraging and making reflection accessible to a group of volunteers, suggested I explore the possibility of my practice as a research project. A few months later, a hospital unit manager asked for my help, saying that staff morale in their team was especially low. Tentatively, I offered to "do some reflective sessions". This, I thought, would combine healthcare professionals and clergy as reflective practitioners. The initial experience consisted of reflective sessions on three occasions lasting no more than half an hour in a meeting room adjacent to their unit, with staff free to attend. On each occasion, groups of five or six staff gathered, and instinctively I opened the session by asking the question I often ask in any pastoral encounter: "How're you doing?" This was meant to be as open as possible and has, then and since, often evoked a revealing response, indicating how the other person is, or is not, coping with their current situation. In this case, the staff in these groups said they were particularly grateful for this space to talk, and their instant relaxation was palpable.

My desire has been to make a difference to the healthcare professionals (HCPs) amongst whom I work by exploring how reflective practice may help with their stress and low morale. I want to aid their own discovery of the resource of an inner sanctuary. This means making use of and developing both the intuitive-personal and trained-professional reflective space. It is my desire to empower others. This is as a priest alongside them as one who identifies places of change and transformation in oneself and others. I want to help them find their voice within their own particular story. My professional practice has grown with this research and has changed part of the culture of my own department significantly, within my work and the language we use. Within both institutions of healthcare and the Church, I have sensed the potential for developing self-exploration and self-awareness by reflection. This research involves finding a voice for the voiceless, self-empowering and strengthening, and self as a source of discovery and healing.

The professional doctorate programme provided a framework to explore my practice as a chaplain who encourages reflective skills. As I embarked on this, my first objective was to see how healthcare professionals dealt with the challenges of their day-to-day work. Suspecting that many may find the obligation to use reflective practice for professional development as onerous and frustrating, I wanted to help empower them to make more fulfilling use of this already available skill. To enhance this, I also wanted to find a simple and memorable reflective practice tool readily accessible in the workplace environment that could provide space for wellbeing. Like an inner sanctuary, this device is something to carry within oneself, for one's own nurture. It is also intended to help connect with others on their shared journeying.

The basis for this research journey is in my ontological and epistemological position and these "assumptions" form the basis of the methodology (Mason 2002: 59) for generating knowledge.

## Generating knowledge

Within research are key paradigms or "beliefs" that reveal "a worldview" of the researcher—which are "based on ontological, epistemological and methodological assumptions" (Guba and Lincoln 1994: 107).

I understand my ontology to mean my view of my reality, my view of myself and others, being evidenced and tested in my life. It is then my position in my research (McNiff 2013: 27) and through which my worldview is formed. My ontological position, the "social 'reality'" (Mason 2002: 14) I wanted to research with healthcare professionals, was that knowledge is gained through human experience, people as "living human documents" exploring their stories. This includes them making connections with their own development and that of others. It is my belief that a key part of life fulfilment is made possible from experiencing the immense value of being naturally reflective.

I understood my epistemology to mean the process of knowledge-making that develops me and others (McNiff 2013: 26) and the way I decide what is knowledge (Mason 2002: 16). What I wanted to research, to generate knowledge of, was the process of learning from experience as expressed in reflective practice, demonstrating deeper awareness of self and others. This has developed through lifelong experiences of intuitively processing my own narrative. These reflective instincts have been identified, framed, developed and shared, through a career in nursing, then through ordination discernment, on to priestly and then chaplaincy ministry. Through personal journeying and professional practice, I see reflection as an internal self-help tool for both survival and growth. However, in both my professions, I have seen reflective practice taught, and expected to be used, but neither nurtured nor lived.

This was a key element to the inspiration for this research. When asked to help with staff morale, I offered to facilitate reflective practice for small groups of staff. Continuing to experience it as a source of liberation and learning for myself, I passionately want to empower others to find whatever may be *their own* discoveries through reflection. In the context of my professional practice, the research project was framed in order to learn whether this would be desirable and possible for the nurture of wellbeing for HCPs.

From this, my methodology (or "how we do things", "a journey where we find things out as we go" (McNiff 2013: 27)) was a process of exploring the use of reflective practice for wellbeing. I was exploring the potential for its development within the work environment of HCPs. In this context, this is the development of reflective skills to nurture wellbeing for the individual and their team. By reflecting with others, we create the space for shared learning. This is a way in which I continue to learn. The reflective space is also a place for respecting our shared humanity and for bringing an openness to learn from each other. My research is an example of "knowledge (as) a living process" as we "generate (our) own knowledge from (our) experiences of living and learning" (McNiff 2013: 29). This has been *my* experience throughout my research project and continues to be so in every shared reflective space with HCPs, and also with chaplains and pastoral visitors. Thus, the project methodology involved devising the means of creating such reflective spaces. Knowledge was generated through the collaborative work of chaplain and HCPs, respectively as researcher and co-researchers. We were discovering together and then creating and constructing together.

## Methodology

In my action research, knowledge was generated with ethnographic participation observation over a year, as chaplain reflecting together with healthcare professionals. This means that we were in "a partnership, a process, a conversation, a way of knowing" (Cameron, Bhatti, Duce, Sweeney and Watkins 2010: 36) as people who together, as co-researchers, wanted to find a solution in our particular context. This knowledge was, and remains, primarily for the people involved, but is also of value for others elsewhere. Reflecting now on our *Creating Space* story, I see that a similar process continues as our department story unfolds, working and reflecting together as a team.

From my initial research proposal, I was aware of being a participant observer of my own professional practice and in its development with HCPs. This meant living and working in relationship over time with the HCPs as my data source. I had understood it to be a "strategy" with a sense of "legitimacy" through being there (Aull Davies 2008: 77, 78). This links too with the chaplain's role of "being there" (Speck 1988) meaning being present or "being with" (Wells 2017: 7), so being alongside. The chaplain has a regular practice of being a participant observer, the "non-anxious presence" (Newell cited in Mowat et al. 2013: 39), with a relaxed openness, quietly alert to one's surroundings. I had seen and developed this in the pastoral encounter, in creating space for the other to tell their story, as the skills of the chaplain. This I have developed in this research project, reflecting on the image of chaplain as the "welcoming guest" (Walton, M. 2012: 226), in other words as both host and guest in the pastoral encounter. These images were explored in Chapter 1.

Being a participant observer involves "long term personal involvement" but with participation as the "means of facilitating observation of particular behaviours ... enabling more open and meaningful discussions" (Aull Davies 2008: 81). This sense of ongoing, relaxed, informal conversations is precisely the "listening and prompting" that I shared in the reflective practice workshops (RPWs) of my research project (which will be described later in this chapter). It also involves considering, and constantly reviewing, being either or both participant and/or observer, where observing is key but in a "dialectical spiral", observing in order to see more and develop how to participate (Rabinow 1977, cited in Aull Davies 2008: 81).

I have come to see "participant observation" as more helpfully described as "ethnographic participation" (Emerson, Fretz and Shaw 2011: 2). The closeness of the contact and relationship with those amongst whom the researcher is researching is both my experience in professional practice and in my research project. I value the sense of "immersion... access to the fluidity of others' lives", developing a deeper understanding through "being with other people ... and experiencing for oneself" their context and influences (Emerson et al. 2011: 3). Being involved, however, does not mean that I ceased to be a chaplain, neither did I become a healthcare professional in their field, not "a member in the same sense" (Emerson et al. 2011: 5). However, working together in this way is similar to the multidisciplinary team in healthcare, where the presence and skills of the other contributors are recognized as both equal and diverse.

Working together as co-researchers, I had to be mindful of reflexivity which carefully considers the place of the "researcher" with "the researched in their context" and traditionally is concerned with rigid anxiety about any influence of the researcher (Hammersley and Atkinson 2007: 13). However, research cannot be done "in some autonomous realm ... insulated from the wider society and from the biography of the researcher" (Hammersley and Atkinson 2007: 15). Reflexivity as a central feature of ethnography means living with a constant awareness of one's presence within the research project group. It means acknowledging "that we are part of the social world we study" (Hammersley and Atkinson 2007: 18), in our sharing and also our observation of the world around us.

If I am exploring my view that knowledge is gained through human experience (my ontology) and then wanting to research or generate knowledge in the process of learning from experience as expressed in reflective practice (my epistemology), in the context of the HCPs of my workplace, I believe that I cannot avoid being part of this research. However, if the knowledge we create is to be credible I must identify and make visible my presence there. So, what of my place, then, within this project?

I am interested in empowering HCPs to explore and develop their use of reflective practice for themselves. I am exploring their practice and my practice with them. This is not so much for their professional growth but to see if their existing awareness about reflective practice could be developed for nurturing their wellbeing. In any pastoral encounter, I believe a chaplain, with a patient or member of staff, for example, would have no agenda save for empowering the other to tell their story. This is by listening and prompting, making connections, being alongside while the other person discerns their solutions. In my ethnographic research, knowledge is found in the same way, the HCPs as the "other person" in this reflective encounter. In researching, my "primary goal must always be to produce knowledge" and to "minimize any distortion of [my] findings" that may come from my own views and hopes (Hammersley and Atkinson 2007: 18). In the pastoral encounter with a patient, to offer my solution would be detrimental, because this would be informed by my story and not theirs. In the same way, in the project RPWs, as will be shown in exploring the use of field notes, I need to distinguish between my presence and that of the HCPs. While I cannot separate myself from my ontology and epistemology, I need to be aware of it in this objective, self-observational way that is "reflexivity": "We act in the social world and yet are able to reflect upon ourselves and our actions as objects in that world" (Hammersley and Atkinson 2007: 18).

Ethnography, with its key element of reflexivity, is living learning, an ongoing journey of discovery. This is the essence of the RPWs within and beyond my research project, where the contextual reflection and self-observation on the issues discussed are part of the learning. It is true throughout the period of research as a living process, where the research design is also a "reflexive process" (Hammersley and Atkinson 2007: 21). It also remains true in terms of the development of our chaplaincy team.

Once again, as in my understanding of chaplaincy, my role is "being alongside them as they work out the answers for themselves" (Orchard in Swift 2009: 175). It is a role that constantly re-checks whose story is being told. Reflexivity is an ongoing, living experience, requiring constant self-observation and reflection. Ethnography is a process of living and learning that creates today's knowledge. Therefore, we can only know what we know now, but as living learning it is an ongoing journey of discovery.

In my research project, my field notes were part of the living learning that is ethnography and just as real as the events that produced them (Emerson et al. 2011: 245), a "record of that experienced reality" (Emerson et al. 2011: 245), our experience of the shared reflective space. Thus "ethnographic participation" (Emerson et al. 2011: 2) is a more congruent way of describing the researcher alongside the people amongst whom they are researching. The physical presence of field notes, with the HCPs' reflections and my annotations, are an image of the reflexivity of the project. As I used field notes in my project, we use a whiteboard in our department reflections. In both scenarios, we are reflecting together, both identifiably present on the same page. As genuinely and as openly as possible, this is *our* story.

I will now show the next steps on the journey of my methodology, from the invitation to the audit study, to the pilot study, and then to the research project.

## Method and tools

### Invitation to audit study

The inspiration for my research project started with the initial invitation to help with staff morale on one ward/unit in May 2010. Following this, having provided the first few reflective sessions, I discussed with a more senior HCP whether I could pursue this both on that particular ward/unit and elsewhere in the hospital. She was very encouraging and from her clinical management position also wanted to know what forms of reflective practice may already be taking place across the hospital. At this point, reflective practice was beginning to be used as part of staff appraisals. By means of internal communication (generic email and information notices), we invited staff to tell us what, if any, reflective tools they were using and for what purpose. At the same time another member of staff, in occupational health, had been asked to try to create ward/unit team-building group sessions. The three of us met periodically as the Reflective Practice Forum (2010-11), inviting staff to join us if they were interested in reflective practice, wanting to share or enhance their experiences. This forum met for only a few months having achieved its initial aim, learning that reflective practice was being used mostly for professional development, debriefing after an incident or appraisals. The team-building work was short-lived due to poor response and the re-deployment of the particular member of staff involved.

During this time, I had an increasing interest in wanting to know how much "reflective practice" was being used at the grass roots level, either by individual staff or within teams of HCPs actually on wards/units. This was both *my* contribution to the Reflective Practice Forum and the pursuance of my increasing sense that reflective practice could be used for *more* than professional development in healthcare staff.

### "How're you doing?" Audit (May 2010–December 2011)

The audit, and its development into my pilot study, explored the experience and perception of reflective practice in ward/unit teams of a mixture of HCPs. The audit of this practice was the early work that aimed to introduce the idea of having a reflective session at ward/unit level, and discover the teams' interest, in as wide a field as possible across the hospital. The purpose of this was to gather an overview of the understanding and use of reflective practice by the hospital's HCPs.

In the 2010–11 audit, with very little research knowledge, the recruiting was random and based on any interest expressed by ward/unit/team managers or staff as I visited their units. In time, this included what I now understand to be snowball sampling in terms of "personal recommendations" (Sturgis 2008: 180) as individual staff became aware of my work and invited me to provide reflective sessions on *their* ward/unit.

This random recruiting involved informally approaching individual HCP ward/unit managers while on my daily, routine patient visits, and offering reflective sessions to their team. These sessions I called "How're you doing?", based on my frequently used opening question in many pastoral encounters and the way I had opened the very first sessions in 2010.

With those who expressed an interest I arranged a single reflective session for a time agreed with the unit, for example for some 13.30 or 15.00, on a day that suited best, related to shift patterns and patient visiting. Several wards/units asked me to run this session twice in order to gather as many of their staff as possible. The session gathered as many HCPs as were available at a time, in a space in the ward/unit, for approximately twenty to thirty minutes. I used a pre- and post-session questionnaire of six questions. In the audit, this included a paragraph to explain that this was an enquiry across the hospital into the general use of reflective practice. (In the pilot study the questionnaire included an explanation of my studies in reflective practice.)

The pre-questions briefly asked for the practitioner's existing knowledge and use of reflective practice and also of their personal means of de-stressing at the end of a shift. There were then six presentation slides, with additional pictures, to offer a simple definition of reflective practice using a man in a mirror, and then a brief exploration of the HCPs' usual de-stress means. Using my five-stage reworded reflective cycle (Figure 1), I offered an introduction to reflection for wellbeing rather than the more familiar professional practice. The post-questions asked the practitioner to identify their usual means of ward/unit communication and staff support methods, for feedback relating to their feelings about how this particular kind of reflective practice, as outlined in my session, might be of benefit to their ward/unit in their particular situation.

The session was very informal, creating an environment for free conversation and open reflection, and included discussion on all the questions raised on the questionnaires. There was no obligation to take part, attendance was at the suggestion of their unit manager, and anyone could leave the session at any time.

I asked the attendees in each case, when completing the form, to remain anonymous by avoiding writing anything that would identify them in name or job. I would have been aware of the ward/unit from which the paper had originated. It was this verbal consent that was understood and approved by the hospital's then Chief Nurse for the purposes of including the data in my potential doctoral programme, as well as in a publishable article, and as part of my general practice. It was also the senior nursing staff's desire that the HCPs in their units should develop further the use of reflective practice as part of their work culture.

This was an audit of existing professional practice, exploring awareness of reflective practice at grass roots ward/unit level for HCPs. It invited them to consider whether they would use it for wellbeing for themselves and their team. Although I showed them the five-stage reworded reflective cycle, I was not directly inviting them to use it at that stage. The use of this reflective cycle will be explained under "research proposal".

This exploration of existing practice continued as my pilot study, following the same purpose and format, starting the research process.

## "How are you doing?" Pilot study (January–July 2012)

The pilot study refers to data generated during these dates in 2012, using a revised questionnaire. This incorporated consent, confidentiality and this pilot as an early stage in my doctoral research process. In all other ways, the study followed the same format as the audit outlined earlier. The process followed the same sampling as wards/units became aware of my studies and expressed interest. It also followed the same arrangements for timing and arranging sessions. It continued to develop across a wider number of wards/units and HCPs, to twenty-three ward/unit teams and over two hundred HCPs. The most significant contribution of the pilot study was in developing my awareness of the research process.

# Becoming a reflective practitioner

## The reflective cycle

Adopt change of practice → Event or experience → Identify and examine issues → Reflection: what should I learn? → How will this affect my practice? → (Adopt change of practice)

### Professional practice

## "How am I doing"—my review of the day

The day's activities and moods? → Good bits? Bad bits? → What can I "see"? Making connections, noticing, discovering… → Anything personal? What have I learnt about myself and others? → Anything I need to do? → (The day's activities and moods?)

### Wellbeing

## Conclusions after the pilot study (July 2012)

Both the audit and pilot study, differentiated by adjustments to the questionnaire and dates used, revealed identical data. Over fifty per cent of the HCPs had received training in reflective practice, but only eleven per cent of those could recall any detail. They described an existing "coffee room culture" in which most positively valued space to talk, even if just a brief opportunity to chat with colleagues. This linked with their common practice of thinking things through on the way home and talking to a partner or friend. Together this affirmed that there was room for further exploration and potential development for a cultural shift to use reflective practice individually and for their team. The outline of the audit and pilot study then formed the basis for planning the research project methodology.

The challenges required flexibility in time and space. The consistent risk related to the practicalities of gathering staff together in the face of their work pressures. Shortage of staffing numbers or sudden ward/unit changes were examples of reflective groups being cancelled at the last minute and alternative times arranged.

## The research project

### The next step—data generation April 2013–April 2014

Building on the audit and pilot studies, I extended the fieldwork in the same hospital for the research project to include eight HCP ward/unit teams (over 150 HCPs). Having received ethical approval for my research proposal from both the supporting university and the hospital's Research and Development department, the fieldwork for the research project began in April 2013 and data generation followed for a year until April 2014.

**Figure 1:** *A development of the reflective cycle from those most familiar for professional development and education (e.g. The Reflective Cycle (adapted from Gibbs, Farmer and Eastcott 1988) and Kolb (1984) as cited in Bulman and Schutz 2008: 225) to my reworded cycle for wellbeing included in the research proposal.*

## Methods for the research project

### Reflective Practice Workshops (RPWs)—recruiting and sampling

In order to include a wide number of HCPs, through purposive or theoretical sampling to fulfil the research question (Mason 2002: 129), I initially recruited six diverse wards/units to include non-nurse and non-ward-based HCPs. This was by contact with their ward/unit managers. This increased to eight teams at the request of senior staff to include two particular units. The sampling number seemed realistic both in terms of running reflective groups on a regular diarized basis and over a period of time. In reality, the majority of teams self-selected, several desirous of following on from the pilot study, asking to continue or join. This also self-generated the diversity of the sort of HCP grouping. In part for anonymizing the teams, as well as ensuring sufficient diversity, I wanted to avoid using solely nurses, and so committed to calling the data source "HCPs" and ensuring that the sampling included at least three different professional groups and some mixed teams. This also seemed to happen naturally.

I generated data from participant observation, or "ethnographic participation", as a means of "being with other people... and experiencing for oneself" their context and influences (Emerson et al. 2011: 2, 3). My use of field notes was as a "record of that experienced reality" (Emerson et al. 2011: 245). This was within the RPWs, using my reworded reflective cycle. Initially, as facilitator I also aimed to identify those willing to lead as the groups developed (noting facilitator skills taken from, for example, Moon 1999, and Bolton 2010, and subsequently from NHS facilitator training 2014). This was to explore whether as the practice developed, they might wish, and feel able, to self-lead and self-sustain the reflective practice.

At each session the attendees, voluntarily drawn from staff on duty on that ward/unit on the day of the reflective session, were likely to vary because of shift patterns, but each were cared for under the same ethical measures employed throughout. This variability represented the same flexibility of the daily challenge of staffing numbers, important if reflective practice is to become part of their working culture.

### Five-stage reworded reflective cycle (2010–13)

The audit and pilot study demonstrated an amalgam of familiar reflective cycles in order to establish the existing awareness of reflective practice among the data source HCPs. I had wanted to adapt the cycle to use words at each stage, from event exploration to more personal or wellbeing reflections rather than to professional practice. In order to express this, I described it as "How're you doing? My review of my day". From the outset, from the audit, I described it simply as a "reworded cycle". The initial five-stage, reworded cycle (Figure 1) asked these questions, allowing for discussion:

- The day's/week's activities and moods?
- The good bits and bad bits?
- What can I "see"? Making connections, noticing, discovering...?
- Anything personal? (What have I learnt about me? About others?)
- Anything I need to do/follow up in any way?

It aimed to keep to the five familiar stages (event, issues, reflection/learning, change and adaption) but rather than picking over any one event or experience, the stages are opened out, with rather more fluid questions, to invite both conversation and exploration of the effect on oneself over the time period being reflected upon. The emphasis is on self-awareness, with the intention to prompt personal reflection, a review of one's day or recent period of time. This, I have suggested, could be used as a personal debrief on the journey home at the end of a shift and also as a tool for group reflection as a ward/unit team, ideally daily but certainly regularly.

The first stage of the cycle explores feelings and moods through the activities of the day or week, identifying whatever the issues may be, how individuals or the team have been over recent days or how they would describe themselves or their experiences. Secondly, anyone may express thoughts on what has been positive or felt good from the day and *only then* to move on to reflect on the potentially negative, any issues that weigh on one's mind as not good or successful.

The third stage encourages insight, noticing what one can "see", making connections, reflecting on any sense of discovery, perhaps gaining a better understanding of reasons for an action, behaviour, use of skills or coping strategy. This brings the opportunity to speak freely to one another about shared noticing by looking, identifying wellbeing or unease.

The fourth stage invites thoughts on personal development from those situations, learning about oneself and others. The fifth stage explores what may need to be acknowledged as a source for further reflections in any way.

This reflective process follows the pattern of well-known cycles, opening the issues with dialogue. However, it focusses organically on the participant's inner self and wellbeing, drawing out insight and possible conclusions. This self-awareness process encourages exploring a more *personal* perspective in coping with the work challenges in both a reflective and reflexive way. It means not only learning from the experience but also being able to identify change in oneself (Bolton 2010: 14). It can also develop a more open forum for team communication and team-building, including identifying skills and issues in and for one another. It draws from the *function* of theological reflection, which seeks awareness of self in connection with the transcendent. Here, using a reflective cycle in a more personal way encourages a sense of self exploration, potentially also nurturing team cohesion. It creates a space for asking one other, "How're you, or we, doing?"

**A vignette—March 2013**

This first vignette is an example of an RPW using my initial five-stage cycle in order to provide a more visible image of these events.

"How're you doing?" I gently asked with a smile and slowly looking around the room. Five healthcare staff had come from their unit into the side room for a reflective session with me during the early afternoon, just before the visitors were due to arrive. Their body language said it all, with shoulders drooping down and torsos slumped, as they almost fell into the chairs. The conversation continued as they described the busy morning, someone off sick making the staffing numbers difficult on a heavy unit, and the tension of the non-stop pace. After a while, when it felt as though they had painted the scene of the morning I asked if there had been any "good bits" over the last few days. Someone mentioned a patient who had said thank you, another described his day off, and another spoke about seeing an improvement in one particular patient in recent hours. The discussion continued and after a while I asked, "And any bad bits?" The chatting focussed on staffing issues, expectations of staff's achievement from senior management in spite of heavy challenges, no one ever saying thank you at the end of the shift, and their sheer exhaustion. "Reflecting then, maybe a little more deeply, what can you notice or make connections with, maybe see with further insight?" We talked about the human connection: a recovering long-term patient who liked to hold hands with the staff caring for him, the anxious relative who hugged the doctor ... the links with personal lives and not only professional practice. One member of staff spoke about her personal issues at home. After a while, the reflections drew to a close with a few smiles and plenty of teasing, as the staff night out was being planned for the next weekend. As they left to go back to the unit one of the staff said, "Thank you, you've given me space to feel human again!"

**Four-stage "wellbeing cycle" (from July 2013)**

> "I do like the wellbeing cycle!" Remark from HCP after RPW
> (17 June 2013)

By July 2013, it became clear that a simpler, four-stage cycle had evolved. Each "stage" often easily rolled into the next as the discussion in the workshop developed. For a while, I had wondered about the clarity or accessibility of the wording, especially of the second and third (of five) stages in the cycle. I had noted that the first and second stages often seemed to run into one another, and although my field notes identify them separately, nevertheless my journal notes that the discussions around "the day's activities and moods" either of that day or in recent days (Stage 1), often include the "good bits/bad bits" (Stage 2).

I usually let the conversation flow, albeit recognizing the stages being moved through, gently, almost unobtrusively leading them through rather than strictly moving from one to the next. The reflective cycle was often more of an aide-memoire rather than a fixed-stage process. I called this the "wellbeing cycle", with thanks to the HCP's remark. To make this easily memorable I developed the acronym HELP.

## The four stages

### 1. How's today—lows and highs?
This is introduced by asking in a relaxed, open way for general feelings about today's or recent days' work, to explore a challenging event and something that was more fulfilling or fruitful. This invites story, talking about general feelings of today's work, or of recent shifts or events that come to mind. It may be one event that emerges, or several.

### 2. Exploring—insight and reflection
The reflection may progress to this stage easily, without anyone noticing, but includes exploring the deeper issues of the experience or event(s), the situation or people, reflections on the stories that have emerged. Prompting to move to this stage is only occasionally needed.

### 3. Learning—about me and others
This may be the point where the group needs encouragement to move from the issue to other, deeper learning, through an invitation to consider what has been learnt about oneself and others, or through encouragement to identify where experiences have prompted other thoughts or connections about people and situations.

### 4. Pondering—things to think over
The final stage is the summary, the time to consider what one takes from this reflective session, what one may be left thinking about, what difference having this space for reflection may have given. Particular to context, "From reflecting on today, what will make me better at . . . N . . . tomorrow/next time? What from today will make another day better?"

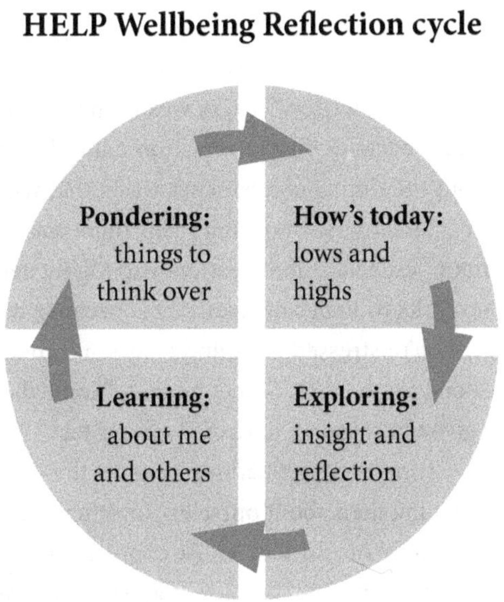

## HELP Wellbeing Reflection cycle

**Pondering:** things to think over

**How's today:** lows and highs

**Learning:** about me and others

**Exploring:** insight and reflection

**Figure 2:** *The "wellbeing cycle" with the acronym "HELP"*

## Reflective Practice Workshops

The workshops consisted of between three and eight participants for approximately twenty to thirty minutes and were arranged monthly (dates, times and venue arranged with the ward/unit manager) for one year, but allowing flexibility to become more frequent if the ward/unit desired.

### A vignette—April 2014

This second vignette is an example of an RPW using my evolved four-stage cycle in order to help provide a more visible image of this practice and to show the development.

"So, how's today?" I asked, as the small group gathered, moving their chairs into the middle of the room, and the general natter subsided. Someone said it was a lovely day but a busy shift, and then the reflections began to emerge with phrases like "keeping each other afloat", which developed into, "It's what it should be like; it's your colleagues that help you!" As the reflections continued there was a lighter feel among them, getting these feelings aired, and one HCP remarked, "Support of each other means you're less stressed." There was no need to invite them to explore this further because the conversation naturally continued into a discussion about the timing of a patient's wash, that while this would be expected to be done in the "morning rush", there was more "space in the early afternoon" especially if the patient was highly dependent. This returned the remarks to issues of stress: "... because it does transfer to the patient if you're stressed ... ", and they continued to reflect on the heavy workload at that time. Someone said, "Some days I doubt the quality of care given because we're rushed off our feet." After a moment or two of quiet, letting these reflections hang in the air, I said gently, "What are we learning then about ourselves or other people?" An HCP said she felt sad because of a patient whose condition was deteriorating, that they had known the patient for a while, as well as her family: "We've bonded; we've connected with her." This feeling of "human connection" continued in their discussion. After a while, and following a quiet moment, I asked, "So what are you left pondering? What do you take from this session?" The replies were clear, saying it had been "somewhere to tip out experiences" and "space to support each other", and they had been "sharing experiences about how to deal with incidents and patients' vulnerability". The final thought was that they had been reflecting on the value of "quality care, not rushed care".

## Facilitating—opening RPWs

Within my ethical care of the data source, the RPWs began with making clear the issues of consent and confidentiality. The two documents, a participant information sheet and a consent form, were given at the start of a session. Thereafter the endeavour was to create a relaxed, informal, conversational atmosphere. Copies of my reflective cycle were on the table or else handed round, depending on the layout of the room.

After general chatting as the group settled, and identifying the time available, I asked, "So, how're you doing? How's today?" The style of reflection was conversational and relaxed, noting the silence but offering space to speak and to listen, as participants wished. As in any pastoral encounter, I saw my facilitating as listening and prompting in order to encourage the other to continue to tell their story.

I decided not to audio- or video-record the RPWs because I thought that the participants may find this prohibiting and intrusive, making them hesitant or constrained in speaking. Someone taking notes is much more familiar in their healthcare work context. While recording is understood to be an efficient method of capturing the mood and the data for transcribing and checking, note-taking is said to be more reflective, helping with a "better yield of analytic themes" (Fielding 2008: 274). Also, recording "can shape the process of ethnographic work" and so will not necessarily be an automatic means of data generation (Hammersley and Atkinson 2007: 147). In trying to create a relaxed and natural space for their reflections, familiar and replicable in style, to have recorded the RPWs would have inhibited this particular research process. For me, electronic recording in this context felt rather false and imposed. There is a physical reality about using a notebook during reflections, noting our contributions, with a real-time quality to it. This includes being able to check back with participants, in that context at that time, at the end of each RPW, that these notes described our reflective group today. This enhanced the participants' voices, empowering them to see and affirm or correct what we had said. My notebook was part of each RPW, with my field notes and not an electronic recording tool. As has been indicated, I was working within each group and not "in some autonomous realm" (Hammersley and Atkinson 2007: 4, 15). The use of field notes was part of the ethnographic research "as a record of that experienced reality" (Emerson et al. 2011: 245), an experience that we shared.

## The reflective community—RPW groups at the end of data generation

My data source has been eight groups of HCPs meeting over a period of a year. As both a data source and as human professionals, the effect on them and the contribution they have made continue to be seen both in their own practice and that of others. Ethnographically they continue to generate data for themselves, in different ways, in the continued use of reflective practice for wellbeing among them and elsewhere.

## Taking a step back? Professional reflexivity

The essential nature of reflexivity in this ethnographic research project has been explored. This differs from, although complements, what I now see as professional reflexivity. This is self-discovery, "thinking from within experiences", "able to stay with personal uncertainty" and "the self they find there" (Bolton 2010: 14, 58).

This research project is an ongoing process of discovery and change, professionally and personally, both in the knowledge created through research and also in my own development. Reflective practice that includes both reflexivity in research work *and* professional reflexivity can be an "ongoing constituent of practice" and "a foundational attitude to life and work" (Bolton 2010: 2, 4). This connects with the chaplain's own sense of daily reflective and reflexive practice, reviewing and learning oneself, and through peer review, about the validity of one's practice, with the pastoral encounter as a source of learning. This is creating space for checking and re-checking one's ability to be the "empty handed" (Swift 2009: 175), "welcoming guest" (Walton, M. 2012: 226). Elsewhere in my thesis, I considered further my own professional reflexivity and professional development. Further reflections on these themes will be seen in our concluding chapter.

Thus far, I have described the steps of my methodology, how my ontology and epistemology are at work here, and how knowledge has been generated through this research. I have explored my action research with ethnographic participation observation, and how reflexivity contributes in, and impacts on, being involved in my research. I have described my audit/pilot studies and the development of the research proposal, outlining the methods and their evolving adjustment. I have shown the steps of data generation, including developing a simple reflective cycle towards nurturing a new holistic, relational, contextual sense of wellbeing for HCPs.

I will now offer a brief outline summary of the generated data from this research and then reflect on the use of the new reflective cycle during and immediately after research.

## Outline summary of the data

Using a simple method of thematic analysis, both as a way of starting to explore qualitative data and as an authentic tool in itself (Braun and Clarke 2006), I noticed seven themes that were revealed over several phases of reviewing the data. This analysis showed in two ways how the HCPs' reflections are consistent with a broader definition of wellbeing than only the institutional "health" model. The first six themes demonstrate the issues on which they reflect—professional concerns, making the human connection between each other and with their patients, issues with patients and relatives, valuing the space to reflect together and expressing the desire for shared team support. These are consistent with the "multi-layered, whole person in relation to their community and context" (Mathews and Izquierdo 2009: 5) as a developed interpretation of wellbeing.

Secondly, by applying a wellbeing characterization tool created by using a summary of definitons, I also re-examined the data against the literature and affirmed the presence of the seventh theme of wellbeing. It is this that the HCPs demonstrate in their reflections, being consistent with wellbeing that includes the holistic, relational and contextual understanding.

Here are real people who, given the space, talk about their experiences, reflect on their stories and share their insights. Through several phases of reviewing the data, the regular shape of the RPW became evident, meaning the issues raised and often the order in which these issues were discussed. The four-stage "HELP wellbeing reflection" process produced these themes—firstly professional concerns, secondly the human connection, thirdly reflecting on valuing their colleagues and lastly celebrating the value of the space to reflect. This reveals the reflections of the whole person, in their relationships and in their context. In both their data, and in the shape of their reflective process, the HCPs show that for them, wellbeing is more than health: that it also relates to the whole person, in relation to others, and in their current context.

Taken from linking the data and wider definitions of wellbeing in the literature, I want to draw attention to the ONS definition I have used. Their four measures noted are "life satisfaction", "feeling what one does in life is worthwhile", "happiness yesterday" and "anxiety yesterday" (ONS 2014: 1, 2), which relate to one's quality of life. They also include looking back, reflecting on one's feelings. In their reflections the professional and human HCPs show that they too seek a quality of life. Connecting with a national data source, I invite those in healthcare to see wellbeing of HCPs as a national concern.

By drawing together the themes, I demonstrated the implication of the broader understanding of wellbeing and then, exploring the process, argued for the value of healthcare professionals' development of a reflective process to nurture this. Having shown the significance of this for HCPs, I will explore the process of using my HELP reflective model, arguing for its use towards developing reflective practice to nurture this new wellbeing understanding.

## Reflecting on the HELP Wellbeing Reflection Cycle

Building on work in experiential learning (Dewey 1933; Kolb 1984), my HELP Wellbeing Reflection Cycle develops the use of reflective practice in both a professional and personal way. I build on Kolb's view of the learning process that combines work development and personal integrity (Kolb 1984: 225). My reflective process also develops connections with the whole person, linking "life situations" (Kolb 1984: 33). As an original model, and using it for wellbeing rather than for developing clinical practice, the HELP cycle advances the combination of work and self. The emphasis, however, is on learning for personal and shared wellbeing in the work environment, through an increasing sense of self-awareness. It is a process, rather than a testing of new knowledge, that serves as a step for leaving the reflective space empowered with a greater sense of wellbeing.

This is a change in professional practice for HCPs and chaplains as co-reflectors. It is *not* supervision. While other forms of reflection are evident in certain parts of healthcare, this research project works towards developing the practice further with groups of ward/unit HCPs in their own familiar team and specific environment. This works towards reflective practice as a personal development tool through building space and as an evolving culture. It includes the increased trust in small, familiar teams; wellbeing seen in relationship and support; giving voice to one another; and learning from experience in oneself and together as a team.

This research further developed Kolb's (1984) work with the clarity and memorable nature of the four-stage model, inviting self-awareness in the process of nurturing wellbeing through reflection-in-action. As detailed in the methodology, by three months into data generation, it was clear that the five-stage reflective cycle had evolved into a simpler, four-stage process. Here each "stage" often easily rolled into the next as the discussion in the RPW developed (Figure 2). Also at each stage the words evolved into simple, memorable phrases. Over time it was often more of an aide-memoire rather than a fixed-stage process. With thanks to the HCP who called it the "wellbeing cycle", I soon after developed the appropriate acronym "HELP", so it became the HELP Wellbeing Reflection Cycle. If the culture of reflective practice in healthcare is to develop, then the reflective model needs to be simple, memorable and apposite for frequent use. Like an inner sanctuary, it needs to be carried within. As I considered an acronym, it began with the "highs and lows" of Stage 1 that had evolved in May to July 2013, and then "exploring" and "learning" easily fell into place. The "pondering" came instinctively from these famous reflections: "Mary treasured all these words and pondered them in her heart" (Luke 2:19). The HELP acronym seemed apposite for a wellbeing reflective resource. Simple, clear and memorable, used frequently, it becomes a tool for life. The continued evolving use of this reflective cycle will be evident throughout our "creating space" story.

## Self-supporting space

Encouraging the HCPs, in time, to self-facilitate their own reflective groups was also a contribution to reflective practice, healthcare and the chaplain's role. Two of the eight groups in this project have regularly been involved in self-facilitating, and subsequent to the project, other existing and new hospital and external groups are developing this.

## "Reflection-in-action" (Schön 1983)

This reflective practice research project responds to and develops Rolfe's (2014) call to return to Schön's "reflection-in-action" (1983). This means that HCPs "reflect on-the-spot, in the here-and-now, and the products of their reflections are immediately put into practice in a continuous and spontaneous interplay between thinking and doing, in which ideas are formulated, tested and revised" (Rolfe 2014: 1180). While Rolfe has the development of professional practice as the original intention, I have developed this in a reflective process to nurture the wider holistic, relational and contextual sense of wellbeing.

Reflecting in the moment explores the human experience as it is known, at this point in time, making initial processing possible. Combining the human and the professional, at this moment, it allows for reflecting with those involved, colleagues on duty at the time and in this situation. It also provides the basis for later reflection once the initial thinking has given room to deal with today's challenge. The potential for spontaneity means issues are likely to be explored in their immediacy, relieving the pressure that a challenge may have brought.

This kind of reflection guides reflective practice towards becoming a more visible feature of daily working life and practice. This makes it increasingly evident in the work culture and a source for self-discovery for those using my research model now. By becoming part of the culture, this may also engender a more natural, less onerous practice of reflection for professional development.

Evidence of the evolving nature of this reflective space continues to develop in a variety of contexts, introducing people to a simple but structured process. The continued evolving use of this reflective cycle will be described in terms of its use in the hospital healthcare professional environment but also in a variety of other ways with chaplains and in other contexts, in this *Creating Space* story of our evolving practice.

## From sluice to classroom to office to... a variety of contexts

*"Are you still doing your reflective stuff?" Healthcare professional, corridor (March 2016)*

In the three years that lapsed between data generation (2013–14) and final submission (2017), I was able to observe any cultural shift or influence affected by this research. These were identified as following themes of teaching, staff support, working with new, reflective teams and the effect on our own chaplaincy department.

## Teaching

From very early on in my research, I was invited either by the local university or professional development tutors to teach reflective practice to a variety of HCPs, going from NVQ to Diploma, Degree and Master's levels. Initially, I taught an introduction to reflective practice combined with holistic care of the patient and oneself (to healthcare assistants) and this developed in several areas, combining reflective practice with other subjects for registered HCPs. These included reflection as part of exploring spirituality and religion, self-awareness and wellbeing themes, and a variety of "end-of-life" and bereavement training.

As a result of my doctoral study programme, since 2011 I have offered two distinct study days on several occasions for diocesan and local clergy. The first was "Practical Theology in the Acute Hospital Context", which explores the reality of healthcare ministry, to aid reflection on their pastoral and spiritual care (parish or elsewhere) and offer a fresh understanding of our shared ministries in the light of today's study of practical theology. This evolved into, in addition, a half day for curates, introducing them to hospital visiting, the profession of healthcare chaplaincy and the distinction between pastoral care as a parish priest and as a chaplain.

I was also invited to support one of the healthcare professionals now required to show evidence of using reflective practice as part of their registration re-validation. For them, I designed a study session with a re-familiarization with reflective practice and the use of my HELP reflective cycle and group support. Other teaching has included medical students, initially an annual session as a special studies unit exploring spirituality, which I developed into the study of spirituality, holistic care and reflection.

## Staff support

Our practice of regularly seeing staff one-to-one for reflection and also facilitating staff teams' reflection has provided two distinct and regular means of staff support in connection with this reflective research. The reflective practice research has been both the means and the tool by which this has developed. This has been through growing awareness across my data source and across the hospital, either directly from the teams/units involved, or from HCPs or different levels of management. The actual practice of reflection using my HELP Wellbeing Reflection Cycle has become my usual reflection tool, either literally or as an aide-memoire, and has grown to be used in several wards/units in their own way and timing pattern or else inviting me or a colleague to attend in the event of a particular subject need or after an event or crisis. There is a distinct culture now of either a regular pattern of reflective practice sessions or single event-based sessions using reflection as a means of staff support. The development of this, now known as "Space for Wellbeing", is described further in a later chapter.

## Beyond the first teams

The wider response to my professional use of reflective practice with HCPs, and the specific use of the HELP Wellbeing Reflection Cycle, has gone well beyond the initial teams. Distinct examples reveal the image of the chaplain as "reflective companion". These include a team that had gone through a very stressful period of time that also involved staff bereavement, and another team that had experienced a series of challenging events in both clinical practice and for its team members; both teams invited me to meet with them on several occasions. Other teams have invited us after so-called "never" events, or distinct individual or team crises, or a distressing, albeit routine occurrence. These have been either urgent calls to set up a reflective session now, today, or else to plan one or several in advance. Several ward/unit teams, hearing of my research and deciding that their morale could be helped with reflection, have asked me to help them use it. We have met in teaching rooms, in a variety of offices, round desks, tea-trolleys, clinical rooms, side rooms and ward sluices, to name but a few. Individual staff have asked if they may use the HELP Wellbeing Reflection Cycle elsewhere in their non-work occupations and groups and/or to take it to other professional groups.

From this research, the role and our chaplaincy team's link with occupational health has developed in two ways. From the early stage of the data generation, the now operational group for "staff health and wellbeing" were supportive of my project, seeing this as part of their portfolio. Further, the chaplains are seen as the "crisis team" in terms of immediate staff support on the ground, being available twenty-four hours a day, offering reflective sessions for wards/units even on an on-call basis. This research has made this both possible and visible.

From 2016–17, invitations to set up RPWs for non-professional and non-clinical healthcare employees have been several and are ongoing.

## Chaplaincy team

Since starting my chaplaincy ministry in this department in 2009, my research project (2010–17) has been a significant backdrop to the cultural shift towards making reflective practice, with my HELP Wellbeing Reflection Cycle, the familiar daily language and method of reflection. It was the initial source of the department's experience of discovery and commitment to the shared journey of learning. Our *Creating Space* story describes how this continues as a combined journey with contributions from every member of the team.

This reflective process is used daily with pastoral visitor volunteers and chaplains in our department at the end of the volunteers' morning visits. This is facilitated by a chaplain, or one of the more experienced volunteers as their ministry develops, but really it is reflection in dialogue following this model or based on this process. As has been outlined, it is the method used regularly with HCPs' reflective groups and in urgent reflective gatherings, and now in a small number of non-clinical staff across the location of the research project. The way in which our chaplaincy team offers reflective practice across the hospital continues to develop based on this model.

In the department's twice-yearly pastoral visitors' training, now called "Creating Space: The Pastoral Encounter", the central focus is reflecting on every aspect of the pastoral encounter. It introduces new volunteers in their pre-practice training to reflective practice as a means of learning and self-development. As the course continues to thrive and develop, regularly reviewed based on constant discoveries, reflective practice is the central tool for learning and the central feature as the course gains attention in local parishes, dioceses and regional conferences, which will be described in a later chapter.

Thus far I have described my own research project, developing reflective practice for the nurture of staff wellbeing, in some detail in order that, just as the rest of the *Creating Space* story, it may be a resource as we share our discoveries. Like any account of methodology, it is hoped that it could be reproduced in a different context for further research. I have outlined the way in which the HELP Wellbeing Reflection Cycle evolved and is used in our own story, similarly, to help others find ways of adopting or adapting in their own situation. I have shared reflections on the way in which this has contributed to our story and evolving practice. This is part of the way I may have contributed to our story just as Jan brings her significant experience in psychotherapy to our work. Together we will now share our discoveries in the way in which our story creatively unfolds.

CHAPTER 4

# What does "being" look like?

This chapter could have been called "what we do". However, we have already been reminded that whilst chaplaincy has previously focussed on "doing", there is now hopefully an increasing emphasis on "being" (Stobert 2020: 77). Equally the earlier model of Speck's (1988) notion of "being there" also resounds with and best describes our ongoing experience as healthcare chaplains. This connects with "being" in two different strands. First, this is as a presence accompanying others, a particular "ministry of presence" and as a "non-anxious presence" (Newell cited in Mowat et al. 2013). Secondly, this connects with "being" as a living or organic learner, one who is always willing to learn, as a "craft" (Bushell 2008: 60), meaning being reflective and reflexive as a "living human document" (Graham 2009: 151), learning through human experience, willing to learn about oneself and one's praxis, listening and reflecting from each new pastoral encounter.

We will now outline further our sense of "being" in terms of pastoral, spiritual and faith care; in our use of reflective practice and nurturing our pastoral visitor volunteers; in the way in which this ministry continues to develop in our wayfarer community and beyond. The themes of pastoral and spiritual care are threads throughout our story and re-appear at different places along the way, so in several chapters and in their own context.

## Pastoral care means listening to the story

Pastoral care, above all, means creating space to listen to someone's story. This is a simple practice and yet it takes a great deal of time and attention to develop this skill in oneself. It is impossible to create space if we attempt to be alongside someone whilst distractingly carrying our own agenda. We might be feeling anxious about getting it right and not making mistakes. We might be already making assumptions about what this person wants and how we can help them. We might feel under pressure to cheer them up or at least provide words of comfort. It is tempting to feel comforted and reassured that we have plenty of tools in our kitbag, spiritual or religious tools, perhaps.

Clearly, there are useful resources like prayers and orders of service for particular occasions but, first and foremost, we need to prepare ourselves and to practise the art of "emptying our hands", a model outlined in Chapter 1. If our hands and our minds are full of assumptions about what this person might require of us, or our primary thoughts are about what we "need to deliver", we have no available space to watch and wait and listen; we may find ourselves being too eager to respond prematurely. It is a common mistake to underestimate the power of real listening. Practising pastoral care in this way teaches us that being listened to by someone who creates the space into which a story can be poured is oftentimes a rare experience. It is in our nature to "fix" things by being too ready to give advice or hopelessly try to propel the speaker into feeling happier. All too often, pastoral care has been interpreted as "doing" rather than "being". In our context, pastoral care is not about practical work, unless listening is categorized as practical. The key in all of this is to realize that listening is not "just listening".

## Spiritual care means being alongside as the storyteller finds their own solution

Spiritual care is a term often used by those who actually mean religious care, but it is worth distinguishing the two as a starting point for the definition we use here. The distinction is based on the premise that every human being has the capacity for being spiritual and having spiritual needs. Conversely, not everyone is religious or has religious needs. Both spirituality and religion point to something "bigger than ourselves" which helps us make sense of life and its purpose. Religion, however, may be better described as a structure, a set of beliefs; a formal or institutional set of teaching, customs and practices inviting belief in (a) God.

We may define spirituality as encompassing any or all of these notions:

- Making sense of who I am in the situation I find myself
- Self-awareness, my inner life and what influences it
- A process, a search for myself in relation to the world
- *May or may not* link with any religion/beliefs
- "How are you doing?" as a simple assessment
- Being "happy in my skin".

Another way of describing this is to be found in the five features of spirituality (Swinton 2001: 25):

- Meaning—*significance of life, purpose*
- Value—*cherished beliefs, truth, precious thought*
- Transcendence—*appreciate "something" beyond self*
- Connecting—*relationship with self, others, environment, possibly an "otherness"*
- Becoming—*self-awareness, unfolding life with reflection.*

Spiritual care for us therefore has come to mean that which helps the person find a solution for themselves, to connect to something bigger than ourselves. Our role as spiritual caregivers is described by Pearce (2018) in this manner: "The chaplain's listening presence *is* the pastoral encounter, with the pastoral care as the focussed listening, and the spiritual care as this space to help the storyteller to listen to themselves."

Our own department also uses this definition. Spirituality is an expression of one's inner life and journeying, in self-awareness, in deep personal needs and in nourishment. Spirituality is both individual and universal, meaning everyone has it, even if unaware of it—but this is not true of religious belief. Spiritual care is also "being present while the other person works it out for him or herself" (Orchard 2000, cited in Swift 2009: 175).

## Faith care (also known as religious care) is offered only if the storyteller seeks it

There is no doubt that chaplains and pastoral visitors alike can and do provide religious care. This may take the form of prayers requested by the storyteller; they may share in bedside Holy Communion, or provide religious articles such as Bibles or rosaries, holding crosses or Qur'an cubes, or anything pertinent to the faith tradition of the patient. It could mean liaising with those of different traditions who can provide appropriate faith care. What is often surprising for some is that this religious care usually accounts for about ten per cent of the total work done by chaplains. The proportion of *religious* care done in out-of-hours work (emergency call-outs in hospital) is normally higher than that done in most daily chaplaincy work because out-of-hours calls are often end-of-life visits when even those who do not profess a faith can often feel that, in these most poignant times, they want "something religious", even if they are unsure of what that may be.

It may be surprising to those unfamiliar with chaplaincy that we do not operate from a position where faith care is the first thing out of our toolbox. In fact, the notion of any kind of toolbox may be utterly inappropriate. This would be contrary to our definition of pastoral care, which is characterized by a refusal to make assumptions about the visit we are about to undertake and a commitment to not be influenced by our own agenda. Clearly, for those who wish to receive religious care, this can be of great comfort when they are experiencing psychological dislocation from their own community and when being a hospital patient prevents them, for example, from attending a funeral (although of course a funeral may not always be a religious event). Above all, we make no assumptions, and we wait to see where the conversation will lead. Our experience time and again is that even if a patient is a church attender, they do not necessarily desire religious care when visited. Their minister, when referring them, may make that assumption, but it is often the case that the patient simply wants a chaplain to listen, rather than offering religious care as a primary focus of the visit.

## Reflective practice and nurturing volunteers

Pastoral visiting, whether undertaken by chaplains or pastoral volunteers, is vitally enhanced by the opportunity to engage in reflective practice after each session of visiting. Kelly goes even one step further than this, stating "pastoral practice not reflected upon is practice that only partially fulfils its potential" (Kelly 2010: 48).

Developing from our daily reflective practice sessions, evolving from our use of the HELP Wellbeing Reflection Cycle, we share these discoveries. So, why do we have such a strong commitment to reflective practice? No one should leave a visiting session without having the opportunity to unload and share any difficult stories or situations that have been encountered. Each pastoral encounter is a source of learning which will inform our next visit and our ongoing practice. Meeting in a group means that we learn not only from our own visits but from those who share in reflective practice. Therefore even if only two people visit that day, our potential for learning has already doubled. We learn vicariously from the visits of others. A sharing of experience is not only an unburdening of difficult stories, but it is a way of nurturing one another in this demanding work. Groups learn to trust one another with their potential dilemmas and feel increasingly safe to "unpick" stories with one another. It is a means of accountability for the safety of patients who are visited and for both the wellbeing and professional practice of chaplains and visitors. It potentially offers a 360-degree peer review, allowing us to constantly appraise and check our practice. There is significant possibility for the capture of qualitative data that not only informs our current team expertise but also feeds into our teaching and training of new visitors. The data to which we refer emerges in two main forms: what the patient says about the visit and what the pastoral visitor says about the visit.

At the start of their visiting experience, some volunteers have been unsure about the value of reflective practice, because it is new to them in this form. It is perhaps not always easy to speak up and admit that some aspect of the visit may have not gone as well as one may have liked. Some new volunteers mistake the session for a chance to simply list several visits they have made, rather than concentrate on one or two visits upon which to reflect. It takes time for visitors to focus on the process of the visit (the theme of the exchange), rather than the content (biographical details and extraneous material). On occasion, when perhaps it has not been entirely clear what we mean by process versus content, we have offered these questions to help consider what may have been the most important parts of the visit that should be discussed in reflective practice:

- Was the geographical area of the patient's home relevant to report? (content)
- Is a description of what the patient was wearing or any other aspect of their appearance relevant? (content)
- Did you need to share with the reflective practice group any historical details of the patient's life? (content)
- Describe how the patient felt and the *essence* of what they shared with you, rather than too much detail. (process)
- Try and encapsulate in summary why your visit was worthwhile (or not) today. (process)

These questions are designed to help understand the difference between process (in which we are wholly interested, and which is the most important part) and content (which needs to be minimal in recounting a visit). It takes time to become comfortable with reflective practice because it is quite a different process from simply recounting a conversation in the way we might do in daily life. When we recount a visit undertaken, we do not use patient names and we refrain from any distinguishing patient detail that might compromise confidentiality.

## The whiteboard

Several years ago, a serendipitous event occurred during a reflective practice session. A volunteer visitor attempted to describe his visit as he tentatively came alongside a patient and gently encouraged the patient to tell their story. The visitor tried to capture this gentle tentativeness and used the words "a dance of humility". This phrase was such a powerful description of how a pastoral visitor might be that we immediately, and without any planning, grabbed a pen and wrote it on the whiteboard in the volunteers' room. The concept and new tool of the "whiteboard" was born, and we have never looked back.

The whiteboard idea emerged unexpectedly and has grown organically ever since as a tool for learning. Sometimes the phrases written are those by volunteers describing their experiences, like the first example of the "dance of humility". Other times volunteers write up a quote from a patient: memorable ones are, "I so enjoyed your visit because you didn't say anything!"; and "I haven't been able to share that with anyone for fifty years."

Weeks may go by when nothing new is written, but the whiteboard is there for all to see on a daily basis. When the board becomes full of phrases and words, we photograph it and make a copy of that photograph, which lives alongside its forerunners in the volunteers' room. The board then gets wiped clean, ready for the next new phrase. This data has been collected since 2016, and it is gratifying that volunteers use it to remind themselves of not only how visits are perceived by patients, but how they or their colleagues have described previous visits. This is important information, which informs our daily practice and shapes our training for new volunteers. We would argue that this data captured from the patients in particular is crucial, because it is not obtained in a formal way, like a questionnaire, where it would be tempting for the patient to respond in ways they might think we want them to respond, an effect known as "social desirability" which is known to bias responses in many questionnaires. In our case, the data is not attributable to a person, and it is not shaped by the patient's desire to please. The whiteboard has, in effect, become our version of "ethnographic participation" (Emerson et al. 2011: 2) as outlined in Sacha's reflective practice research (see Chapter 3). This means that in our department our pastoral visitor volunteers are our co-researchers.

## Nurturing volunteers

It is important to recognize the impact that hearing difficult stories and being alongside those in distress may have on visitors, whether chaplains or volunteers. Although there are already measures in place that are detailed below, we continue to look for ways in which we can nurture those who carry out this work.

### Training

Pastoral visitors do not visit on the hospital wards without first undergoing the departmental training course (which will be outlined in further detail in Chapter 5). All applicants provide two satisfactory references and are interviewed by two chaplains, to help chaplains assess the suitability of the applicant, and to help applicants understand fully the nature of this work and the ethos of the department they might be joining. If successful, the applicant is trained on a twelve-hour pastoral care course (six sessions, each of two hours, over six consecutive weeks). Once training is complete, and all DBS and occupational health checks are clear, each visitor meets with the lead chaplain to further evaluate the mutual fit for both them and the department. During this post-course evaluation, the pastoral visitor agrees which morning of the week would best suit them and the department to do their ward visiting and their start date is arranged.

We have developed and implemented a "pastoral buddy" system. Initially, the new pastoral visitor was assigned time with an experienced honorary (at that time) chaplain whom they shadowed, and then the honorary chaplain in turn shadowed the new trainee on their assigned ward. This was to help them get started as they began to ward visit, and they orientated to the hospital, our department and to their ward. The system has developed to include a pastoral buddy being made available for the three months of their probation, working with them as desired or simply being their "go-to" support if they prefer. This role is currently fulfilled by a chaplain who has moved from being an honorary to an employed chaplain, and whose own story of developing ministry is outlined later in Chapter 8.

In the event that the number on the course makes pastoral buddying practically difficult for one person to manage, the chaplain delegates to an agreed number of other, more experienced pastoral visitors, as part of their development. She liaises with their chaplain mentor (chaplain and pastoral visitor meet annually for review, but any other time for support). She co-mentors where this is thought to be helpful and has her own list of mentees. The pastoral buddy role also has a "rolling" effect, meaning that while it supports new pastoral visitors, it also helps develop other more experienced pastoral visitors, in the spirit of a department committed to shared and continued learning.

Over time, the pastoral visitor volunteers must renew their training every three years, and this is monitored to ensure compliance. Continued membership of the pastoral team is contingent upon this renewal without exception.

**Volunteer mentoring**

The department decided to support its pastoral visitors in additional ways that complemented the provision of reflective practice. Mentoring was a means of providing additional support for each visitor when perhaps they needed to discuss any issues that had arisen for them in greater depth, or those that required more time and space than collective reflective practice could provide. Each volunteer is assigned a mentor, who is a chaplain. No less than once a year, both chaplain and mentee meet to review the work, the progress and the impact of the work on the volunteer. This is a one-to-one session where the mentee can discuss anything at all. If there is difficulty or concern around the work of the volunteer requiring a sensitive conversation, this can be discussed in the privacy of the mentoring session, rather than in the more public setting of group reflective practice.

At the first meeting, the chaplain will introduce the Volunteer Agreement, which sets out expectations the volunteer can have of the chaplain and department. These include details of support and training available to the volunteer. The agreement also sets out the expectations that the chaplains have of the volunteer, for example to report their absences, attend refresher training and adhere to the relevant policies of pastoral care outlined by the department. They must also understand hospital policies such as health and safety, safeguarding, confidentiality and fire evacuation policy.

**Library materials**
The department provides a small library solely for the use of chaplains and volunteers, which contains books on pastoral care, both of a general nature and those covering speciality visiting (end-of-life, for example). In addition, there is a folder of relevant articles on pastoral, spiritual and religious care which is available for volunteers. This is regularly updated, and volunteers are encouraged to read or copy the articles, which may help with their skill development.

**Quiet Days**
Once or twice a year, as resources allow, a Quiet Day is offered to volunteers at no charge. This is off site at a local venue and includes a small amount of input by chaplains, several periods of quiet during the day, and a garden and chapel at the disposal of volunteers, with a shared lunch and either a meditation or time of prayer.

**Collaborative conferences**
Once a year, a day conference is arranged for chaplaincy volunteers from all over the south-west at a local abbey. There is teaching input from a team of chaplains as well as time for quiet contemplation and networking across teams. Conference themes have included End of Life, Mental Health and Self Care. These conferences are discussed in more detail in Chapter 6.

## Taking this work elsewhere

**Intensive Care Unit (ICU) visiting**
Some years ago, a consultant in ICU noticed that relatives of patients in this particular area of the hospital often had to wait for long periods outside the ward before being admitted to seeing a member of their family, which was potentially stressful given the gravity of those patients' medical conditions; these are among the most seriously ill in the hospital.

He suggested that a team of volunteers should support patients' families and offer refreshment to them and a listening ear. A local church set up a small team of volunteers to undertake this work, which was inevitably demanding, and volunteers needed training to do it effectively and to learn to take care of themselves. The Department of Pastoral and Spiritual Care was asked to offer training for this group of volunteers, and eventually the ICU team was brought under the umbrella of that same department. All new applicants to this team were given the full twelve-hour training, like any other pastoral visitor, and were asked to visit on "general" hospital wards for three months before taking up their duties in ICU. They were also given access to reflective practice, which has become a condition of their Volunteer Agreement.

**Patient Experience Committee (PEC)**
The hospital's Patient Experience Committee wanted to find a new way of collecting patient data describing their hospital stay to better understand the actual patient experience. The Department of Pastoral and Spiritual Care was asked to provide training so members of PEC could marry the principles of pastoral care with data collection to try and assess patient experience without the usual use of structured questionnaires. This was to help the PEC committee to listen to the patient, rather than simply collect and generate quantitative data about the quality of food, noise on the ward and other practical issues. The departmental chaplains trained members of PEC in listening skills, committing to visiting without an agenda other than listening, and being a non-anxious presence for the patient. Members were asked to visit simply as a listener, rather than a nurse, patient council member, or any of their usual hospital roles. They were encouraged to listen rather than ask direct questions and to let the patient take them where the patient wanted to go, rather than follow the visitor's lead.

Once their visits were complete, PEC members were invited to participate in reflective practice with chaplains to share in their visiting experience and to understand how to turn the contents of these conversations into data that could be used to improve patient experience. Teaching this method of combining pastoral listening with gathering information relevant to improving the patient experience was an example of how "what we do" can be used not simply as a supportive presence alongside the patient, but also as a tool for hospital staff to learn to listen more deeply to the patient's story, rather than asking them pre-organized questions about specific topics that the PEC members thought might be relevant to patient wellbeing. In this way, we could emphasize to PEC members that the questions we ask can only generate answers to those particular questions and might not reach other issues that are important to patients.

**Medical and nursing students**
As will become increasingly evident throughout our *Creating Space* story, our relationship as chaplains is to an increasingly diverse constituency, as well as to a variety of healthcare staff, but even then in differing ways. In 2013, we inherited from a previous colleague the opportunity to provide a two-week, annual "special studies unit" for medical students. Under their programme of exploring the multi-disciplinary team, and individual professions within this, students were offered this short placement with us to explore our professional practice and to gain a deeper awareness of holistic and spiritual care. Usually a group of up to five medical students chose this study unit, which combined contact time with us, learning about our role and ethos, shadowing bedside visiting, visiting alone a further two or three patients from whom to develop case studies, time for private study and gathering as a group with one or two chaplains for reflection and discussion. At the end of the course, each student was expected to produce a 2000-word report to be marked by us and submitted to the university. This study unit was developed over the following six years, and the learning outcomes evolved to include:

- an understanding of the contribution of spirituality to the care of the whole person
- an understanding of the value of identifying one's own spirituality, self-awareness and self-care
- gaining in confidence to include spiritual care in the professional healthcare environment and multi-disciplinary team.

Overall students were expected to demonstrate an understanding of holism, spirituality and spiritual care. They would explore different models or definitions of spirituality and show the dialectic of the key issues. Having identified its place in healthcare, they would also explore the way in which spiritual care can be offered in the patient context and how this contributes to care of the whole person.

The group of interested students came from a variety of backgrounds and cultures, some of whom had a faith history often related to family expectation, and others who expressed a genuine interest, without agenda, to understand more about the work of the chaplain. Without exception, however, there was each year an overwhelming sense at the end of the study unit that each student had really valued the space and the self-discovery that this opportunity had given them.

Medical students have also joined us in other ways. At the invitation of a palliative care consultant in 2017, medical students on their rotation were offered space to explore additional aspects of palliative and end-of-life care. In term time, once a week for a morning, up to three students have come to shadow a chaplain or experienced pastoral visitor who is visiting patients at this stage. Before the visit, the students are invited to suggest their existing awareness of the chaplain's role and offered our understanding of pastoral and spiritual care. They are also asked to try to prepare for the shadow visiting by not expecting to ask the patient medical questions but to come and simply listen to the patient's story. Once again, without exception, these visits have received incredible feedback from the students, who appreciated the opportunity to watch us at work but also to consider their own developing bedside manner and the way in which to encourage the patients to talk about how they feel. There have been a number of students who feel this experience with us has given them the confidence to sit and listen to the patient first before asking any detailed clinical questions.

On a wider scale, nursing students have self-referred to our department looking for a better understanding of our role, of pastoral and spiritual care, and of our place in a variety of end-of-life contexts. More broadly, encompassing a number of trainee healthcare professionals, we have over a number of years been invited to teach in several areas.

## Teaching elsewhere

As outlined in Chapter 3, Sacha was invited on different occasions by both the local university and professional development tutors to teach reflective practice to a variety of healthcare professionals. This supportive and training relationship with medical and other healthcare professionals is another example of the development of our growing place in the multi-disciplinary team, but also as a profession ourselves that both "fills gaps" but also shares "mutual hospitality" (Walton, M. 2012: 226) in a growing healthcare community.

# Wayfarer community

The Department wanted to develop a better understanding of those who seek our help and who might not be easily or simply be described as patients, staff or relatives; however, that does not mean that a wayfarer cannot be in one of these groups. A typical example might be someone who, without prior warning, comes to our door and wants someone to listen. This may be a one-off visit, or it may start out that way but develop into a series of visits. It may be, but is not often, someone who gets to know us in this way and then may take the step to becoming a volunteer in the department. There have been those who have joined us not necessarily for regular one-to-one visits, but for the Sunday services in the chapel, because it is a safe space in which to worship without too many questions being asked or any demands being made.

Simply put, there were people who turned up wanting to be helped by our department and then often staying around for a time. We began by describing this feature of our work as "wayfarer church", but we changed this name relatively quickly because "church" did not appropriately or fully describe our relationship with such individuals. At this point, therefore, we are using the term "wayfarer community" to describe people who journey with us for a short while. They may move on and never be seen again, but equally they may at a later date arrive again at our door. The important feature of this group of people is that they somehow have indicated to us that they find a sense of home or community with us, and even when they are not physically present with us they find reassurance that we are there, like a place of refuge they may not need today, but they might avail themselves of in a future time of distress. This is not unlike the idea of a monastic community that welcomes guests for a short period; those guests may help out with tasks in that community, or they may not. But they have a temporary home in the sense that our department is a place where they have a guarantee that someone will provide for them a safe listening space and, when they leave, the knowledge that we are there should they choose to return is important and reassuring for them.

**Meet some wayfarer community individuals...**
*Jean is a regular visitor to our department for one-to-one sessions. She reported that the greatest surprise and relief during her first meeting with a chaplain was about the experience of simply being heard, without the listener intruding with their own story, or admonishing her for being too anxious, sad or angry. It was the only time in her life that she could remember being able to speak of her own experiences without being told to cheer up, her misfortune being compared with others', or being given any kind of advice. She tells me that the benefits she experiences from her visits are significant and are worth the distress she suffers in travelling to the hospital. She has described the anxiety she experiences as she gets on a bus to travel in, the surge of people she has to negotiate at the main entrance and the avoidance of lifts to reach our department. "Once I get to the chapel," she says, "I know I only have to walk a little way to your office and I am 'home'. By this I mean I am in your department and people will be kind and receive me just as I am. I could spend all day there because it feels so safe."*

*Carl is a young adult who was repeatedly admitted to the Emergency Department (ED) after a series of suicide attempts and was seen in ED by the chaplain. He then began to meet regularly with the same chaplain on a one-to-one basis to tell his story and to feel supported for a year or more.*

*Terry was in a difficult place in his life and remembered that his friend had been helped a decade earlier by the chaplaincy department. Terry contacted us and came regularly to be supported for his mental health issues. He also began to volunteer with our weekend bed-pushing team to enable hospital patients to attend chapel services.*

*Rowena calls by occasionally to talk with us and now attends our weekly meditation group. She says that our department is supportive, and she feels able to be comfortable and welcomed when she calls to tell us how things are going in her life.*

**Wayfarer staff too . . .**
*Within our lives working within a wayfarer community, our time alongside individual members of staff or several from a ward/unit team is significant. It may be that someone seeks a listening ear and support after a stressful event or period of time, or their manager feels they need some sort of emotional care, perhaps having behaved uncharacteristically today at work or over time. Staff make initial contact with us in a variety of ways: they may approach us directly, or be recommended to seek us, or we are invited by a manager or a colleague to casually approach them carefully at work, or else they may bump into us in the corridor and start to talk. Indeed, these are small examples of the many ways in which we are very much involved in staff support. The individual, or group, may see us once or over several weeks or months. One significant reflection from this part of the story is that if, for example, someone talks about a particular work-related stressful issue or experience, this is often only the tip of the iceberg, and there are deeper, more serious issues to explore: perhaps relationship concerns, family worries, past event pain unresolved, bereavement or many other personal rather than professional issues.*

We are privileged to accompany the wayfarer community and they remind us of the significant impact of being alongside and listening without an agenda. Whilst we may look like the providers, they are our teachers, and our work with them continuously informs our practice. In other words, our provision of hospitality becomes yet another source of learning for us.

## What does "being" look like in other departmental work?

It will come as no surprise that as a department we offer regular opportunities for patients, relatives, staff and wayfarers to use the space we create in more formal events such as Sunday services in the chapel (a morning Eucharist and an afternoon Mass), a twice-yearly "Remembering Together" special service for those who have lost babies and children, and other diverse occasions such as staff memorial services, seasonal services at Easter and Christmas and weekday reflections through Advent and Lent. In addition, we offer space in a weekly silent meditation for anyone who wishes to attend. Over time, some of these services have evolved into moments of creating space, rather than formal church services, notably the "Remembering Together" service for bereaved parents. What once was a traditional service with hymns, homily, readings and prayers has now become a shorter, more reflective space with a good deal less words. Names of children are still read out, and parents are invited to light candles and place them on the chapel altar. Music is still played, but rather than delivering more spoken religious material than attenders might be used to, we offer gentle prompting with few words to enable the use of quiet space for a time of remembering and commemorating in ways that parents can own themselves. Similarly, in meditation, we create the space and we do not pay much attention to how many people attend; whatever happens in that space is not ours to command, control or worry over. All in all, whether we are conducting a formal service or event, or facilitating something more "fluid", we continue to be committed to creating space rather than filling it with our assumptions about what we think people need.

Thus far, we have explored what "being" means to us in healthcare chaplaincy, alongside others, learning with and from them. We have unpacked our sense of "being" in pastoral, spiritual and faith care; in developing our volunteers as part of our whole team; and the way in which this spills out into our lives within and for a wayfarer community. We will now demonstrate how this sense of "being" is further revealed in our pastoral training material.

CHAPTER 5

# Creating Space: The Pastoral Encounter

In this chapter, we outline the shape and overall content of the training course that we deliver to our pastoral visitors. As discussed in Chapter 1, it has evolved considerably from its early inception. Two main changes will be evident. The first is that unsurprisingly the training course began as a faith-based course; it used Gospel passages to illustrate key points in pastoral training, and it reflected the likelihood that pastoral visitors in the department largely came from churches. The reason this is unsurprising is that in the early days of the chaplaincy, most referrals and visit requests were from local clergy calling to alert the department to members of their congregation who were hospital patients. At that time, therefore, pastoral visitors were largely correct in assuming that the patients they were going to visit were mostly church members who would want some religious input from the visit. This faith-based theme has changed considerably for two reasons. First, the majority of patients we see now have no religious faith and yet still want to be visited. That has shaped our understanding of what chaplains and pastoral visitors offer during a visit: our primary métier now is being alongside to listen to whatever the patient wants to talk about, and to be supportive in helping the patient make sense of what is happening to them. We support them to identify the spiritual resources of their own that they might draw upon (based on our individual but universal definitions of spiritual care in Chapter 4) and we offer religious care, *but only if asked for or hinted at by the patient*. This transition from a narrow, religious perspective was also reflected in the change of name from Chaplaincy to the Department of Pastoral and Spiritual Care in the early twenty-first century—an evolution not just in our own hospital but in many similar departments elsewhere.

It is important here to answer some of our critics, who believe that the current version of the pastoral training is a move simply founded on political correctness resulting in the erasure of all religious content. Indeed one such critic suggested we have turned the original Pastoral Care training into a completely secular course. We would firmly reject these observations and would reiterate that the training in its current form provides for the pastoral needs of any or all patients in hospital. It is not a question of ignoring faith-based matters; rather, we effectively equip ourselves and our volunteers with understanding and skills in offering pastoral and spiritual care, which are universally applicable and relevant, and religious care only when desired by, and appropriate to, the needs of the patient.

The second main reason for a move away from a Christian-based training course was that we found we were recruiting new pastoral visitors both from different faith backgrounds and from no faith background at all. Emphasis grew on offering pastoral and spiritual care as the primary focus, because religious care was being requested on a much smaller scale. In 2015, the current Pastoral Care course changed its name from Pastoral Care Training to the title "Creating Space: The Pastoral Encounter" to describe more fully what it was that chaplains and pastoral visitors alike were offering. For many years, this course encompassed the detail of how to visit in a hospital setting. It included important detail on infection control, identification of different hospital uniforms and specialisms, and other hospital-specific information.

In time, the course content changed from a focus on this hospital because we were receiving more enquiries from potential applicants who were interested in training for pastoral care in settings other than the hospital. This began in 2016 with applicants who were recruited by outside agencies to visit in care homes. It then further expanded as we invited individuals from parishes and other community settings to take advantage of the training. In its current form, the Pastoral Care course has also attracted students from both sociology and counselling/psychotherapy backgrounds who see both training for and experience of pastoral visiting as a valuable resource in furthering their experience, knowledge and skill base in their future careers. For those applicants who train with us to specifically work in the hospital, we provide hospital-specific information, no longer within the course content, but in a training booklet to which they can refer as they begin and continue their volunteering in the hospital.

We realized that the interest from parishes and elsewhere was not going to be served well by chaplains attempting to train at numerous locations out of hours, so our team developed the idea of training different types of candidates (hospital visitors, parish visitors, students) at one location and in mixed action learning groups. This will be discussed in more detail in Chapter 7.

The course that is described below now takes place twice a year, is based at the hospital and incorporates applicants who will, once trained, work as pastoral visitors in their own setting. The content is therefore much more applicable to a wider group of trainees and encompasses case studies and examples not just from hospital visiting, but also from scenarios based on care homes, parishes and other settings. Whilst throughout our descriptions below, we use the word "patient" to describe the person receiving the visit, this is for simplicity, and it is for the reader to imagine who it is that will be receiving the visit in their own particular context. What follows is a description of each module in turn. While areas of this material are repeated elsewhere in our story, it is encapsulated in this chapter to show how these subjects fit into the overall context of the course. Each module begins with a relevant quotation that introduces a central tenet of the session and continues with its main themes. At the close of each module, a case study is provided that is pertinent to the teaching. We have received positive feedback from trainees about how case studies help to embody and exemplify the nature of each module. We then end the description of each module with a section called "final thoughts" before moving on.

## Module 1: Pastoral Care

> "Pastoral care is the practical embodiment of belief in humanity ... critically sensitive to context and disciplined in its response. As a creative art ... it has the potential for being nourishing, inspiring and transformational" (Cobb 2005: 43).

We begin by describing pastoral care as the listening ear to the richness of humanity. This module helps the applicant to understand what we mean, in our context, by pastoral care. It may be that prior to the training, applicants imagine pastoral care as encompassing all kinds of practical help, but here we focus on the skill of listening, creating space for the patient and simply being alongside without any agenda of our own, or any expectations or assumptions about how this visit will unfold.

At this early stage in the training, we introduce methods of learning, through parables or myths, through our life experience and through what we introduce as reflective practice. We have discovered that by introducing the concept of reflective practice from the very beginning of the course, we are giving applicants the opportunity to use it in every training session, to help them become confident about it by the time they complete the course. By teaching in action learning groups—in this case, groups made up of different visitors (hospital, parish, student)—they are able to have richer and more varied group discussion as they reflect together on their learning from the very beginning of the course.

Once the understanding of pastoral care as being alongside, listening, and without agenda is clear, we then proceed to define spiritual and religious care to highlight the distinctions between these three forms of care. This is very much an initial foray into these distinctions, which will be covered in more detail at a later stage in the training.

### Pastoral care

The main features of pastoral care are the provision of a listening ear, a skill in creating space and meeting people where they are. It demands a dedication to being there and being alongside the patient as a companion who is committed to being aware of their agenda, working at their pace with focussed listening.

**Spiritual care**

Spiritual care is about helping the person make sense of who they are in the situation they find themselves, be that distress, illness or any kind of change in circumstance. It is about encouraging their self-awareness and being able to talk about their inner life and what influences it. It includes an accompaniment in exploring a process or a search for self in relation to the world, which may or may not have links with faith and/or belief. In the majority of cases, spiritual care is offered to people of no faith and begins with a simple "How are you doing?" as a preliminary opening to a spiritual assessment.

**Religious care**

By religion, we mean a formal or institutional set of teaching that invites belief in (a) God. One's own spirituality may or may not include a faith based in a religion, and so it is crucial to be aware of the distinction between spiritual care and the provision of religious needs. Differences will be evident across world faiths and interdenominational differences.

The final phase of Module 1 introduces the trainee to the anatomy of a pastoral encounter in preparation for Module 2. The anatomy of a pastoral encounter begins with the acknowledgement that there is a beginning, middle and an end to this visit. However, we stress that it begins before it begins, as we help trainees to prepare themselves inwardly for their visits before they set out to meet someone. In the process of "creating space", there is a need to listen not only to what is said but also what is unsaid, offering a "non-anxious presence" (Newell cited in Mowat et al. 2013: 39) and being aware of the dangers of assumptions on both the part of the visitor and the visited. Through all of this, the visitor needs to remember to be "empty handed" (Swift 2009: 175), so they can hold the story that is being given to them; to recognize the richness of the other person; and to regard whatever is shared as "holy ground", meaning whatever is precious, sensitive and sacred. Through this, the visitor focusses deeply on what they are hearing and seeing with complete awareness and unhurriedly shapes their response. This anatomy is revisited throughout the course.

**Case study**
*"Are you here to cheer me up?" asked the patient. "No," I said. I sat and listened to his story. He was a farmer, and he talked about how amazing it was to be with nature and animals. He cried and thanked me so much for coming and said, "I am so afraid of the future."*

## Final thoughts

### Reflective companion
"The essence of what (we) offer—generic spiritual listening ... active non-judgemental listening that creates a "dynamic holding space" which the person, the storyteller, can use to talk about the present and to revisit and reinterpret events from the past, and in so doing maintain their story or create new possibilities, even a new sense of hope, for the future" (Kennedy and Stirling, 2013, p. 62, 63).

### The richness of humanity
"There are no ordinary people. You have never talked to a mere mortal. Nations, cultures, arts, civilizations—these are mortal, and their life is to ours as the life of a gnat. But it is immortals whom we joke with, work with, marry, snub and exploit—immortal horrors or everlasting splendours. This does not mean that we are to be perpetually solemn. We must play. But our merriment must be of that kind (and it is, in fact, the merriest kind) which exists between people who have, from the outset, taken each other seriously—no flippancy, no superiority, no presumption" (Lewis, 1942, p. 46).

## Module 2: Exploring the Pastoral Encounter

Throughout this training, we affirm the essence of pastoral care as listening, aiming to re-build this vital contribution to human experience, or as the humourist author Erma Bombeck wrote, "It seemed rather incongruous that in a society of super sophisticated communication, we often suffer from a shortage of listeners" (Bombeck 1978: 249, 250). In exploring this key element in any pastoral encounter, we consider how to listen to ourselves in preparation for listening to others. As we learned in Module 1, each pastoral encounter has a beginning, a middle and an end. In this module, we focus on how to prepare ourselves for a pastoral encounter long before we arrive at the start of a visit; being ready to empty our hands of our own thoughts and preoccupations; creating space in oneself; being ready to hold someone else's story.

> "For only when the chaplain's hands are empty, will wounded people dare to offer their stories and allow their utmost shards of doubt and hope to be handled with love and honoured with insight" (Swift 2009: 175).

We look at ways of launching the encounter, to make it clear who we are and why we are there, noting how language at this introductory point can have a significant and sometimes detrimental influence on the direction of the encounter; for example, using the word "chaplaincy" can make people assume we are there simply to talk about religion. Unlike everyday social exchange, a pastoral encounter should have at its heart the idea of "mutual hospitality", of being a "welcoming guest" with the chaplain or pastoral visitor as "an interested guest, as a stranger in a strange land" but who equally is able "to welcome the stranger ... to host the strange ... " (Walton, M. 2012: 226, 233). In the words of the pastoral visitors' quotes from our whiteboard, we are "walking on stage without knowing the plot" as well as "hovering with active gentleness".

We explore what might get in the way of our attempts to offer pastoral and spiritual care and touch on the pitfalls of what hinders a visit, for example our own agenda, interrupting, offering advice, comparing the patient's story with our own experience. These are all human responses of which we are capable in ordinary conversation, but we emphasize how a pastoral encounter is different, because it is not like a simple conversational exchange we might have in the shop or the pub. During each encounter, we ask ourselves again and again, "Whose story is it anyway?" We remind ourselves that the pastoral encounter means we're there to listen; we are not delivering anything, nor are we visiting to cheer someone up. We are there to create space.

**In the middle**
As our focus moves towards the middle of the pastoral encounter, we discuss the importance of non-verbal behaviour for both the visitor and the patient in picking up cues as to each other's perspective in this visit. We discuss the use of silence and its importance in giving space to and honouring what is being said. We also talk about the use of touch. Some trainees worry that because they are naturally people who take someone's hand or place their hand on a shoulder in times of distress, they might revert to this indiscriminately during a difficult or sad pastoral encounter. Some trainees adopt the erroneous notion that we teach "never to touch", but this is not true. What we emphasize is that if touch is used, it must be with a great deal of caution, because some patients may prefer not to be touched for a variety of reasons.

At this early stage, the training introduces the issue of confidentiality and explains that whatever is discussed in the encounter (or even that the visit has taken place) is confidential, unless the person visited has given permission for the visitor to share that information. This is discussed in the light of safeguarding principles, explaining that there is a legal need to share when one is told about issues of active abuse, self-harm and/or harm to others. It is emphasized that the pastoral visitor's response is to alert the teller that other authorities need to know and to inform their leader or the co-ordinator of the pastoral team (chaplain, clergy, care home manager, supervisor).

**Shall I stay or go?**
We need to ask ourselves the following questions. How long is a good visit? How will I know when to leave and how do I leave? What do I want to "achieve" in my visit, and how can I ensure the time spent is worthwhile?

I need to remember that I am meeting people where they are, and I need to ponder on the usefulness of presence and of absence. In other words, I need to be alert to when leaving is more appropriate than staying.

Creating space is about "being with", which builds on the contribution of Samuel Wells (2017) and his distinction between "for" and "with" and "working" and "being" to emphasize the importance of "being with" in a pastoral encounter. We are grateful that these distinctions have helped us and our trainees to reflect on examples of "being" and "doing" in everyday life, in order to understand the importance of "being with" in the pastoral encounter. Finally, we remind ourselves that each pastoral encounter has so much to teach, and the practice has even greater potential by reflecting on it (Kelly 2010: 48).

**Case study**
*"What's that badge you're wearing?" asked a patient of the ward visitor, who explained she was a volunteer in pastoral and spiritual care. "I don't want to talk about religion," said the patient, gruffly. The visitor replied "I'm here just to see how you're doing". The patient agreed the visitor could sit down, and he began to talk about a particular favourite book he loved. He talked and joked and even tried to imagine what sort of books the visitor would like, trying to guess the right sort of books she would read.*

## Final thoughts

To illustrate the exploration of a pastoral encounter, with reflective practice, the "whiteboard" (described in Chapter 4) is introduced. Quotes from the whiteboard are given to show the feedback *from patients* following visits by pastoral volunteers.

"It's MY story. Thank you for allowing me to see me."
"Everyone has a story if someone is willing to listen."
"If you had not come today, this would still be inside me."
"You listening to my story is such a release."

## Module 3: Real Listening

> "Compassion asks us to go where it hurts, to enter into the places of pain, to share in brokenness, fear, confusion and anguish. Compassion means full immersion in the condition of being human" (Nouwen, McNeill and Morrison 2008: 3, 4).

The overall aims of this module are to show how we create space for the patient to tell their story; to recognize when we are too self-referent and to learn how to deal with distractions and barriers (internal and external).

It is only human to be distracted and to pay attention to oneself, rather than really listen to what the patient is saying. But this may mean that we find we are in danger of telling our own story, or being guided by our moods, feelings and fears. We may notice that we are responding with our own views or agenda. Finally, we need to avoid demonstrating that we need to be elsewhere. In the pastoral encounter, the emphasis is on listening and not being tempted to be self-referent. There is a fine line between identifying with the person, making connections and overdoing it by telling our own story. Real listening is central to pastoral care: it follows and prompts the other person's agenda and, regardless of topic, may be "where they are at the moment" or a preamble to more of their story if they choose to share it.

To reinforce the importance of real listening, trainees are introduced to Carl Rogers' three core conditions that are central to person-centred counselling (Rogers 1959). The first condition is "unconditional positive regard", which may be described as a listening without judgement, a valuing of the person in front of you. The second condition, "empathy", is the sensitivity towards and willingness to understand another human being who speaks from their own perspective. The third condition is "congruence", which denotes genuineness and being real. These three terms are from Carl Rogers' "necessary and sufficient conditions" for support, change and/or internal awareness. They are reflected in our experience from pastoral encounters and in the feedback we receive from those we visit; we find that using these terms helps trainees to appreciate how these terms, borrowed from counselling theory, enable us to be better listeners.

Real listening can be challenged by various external interruptions or "noises off", like someone else arriving or joining in a bit too much. There might be distracting TV or radio, or other noises in the environment. There will also be internal interruptions inside the listener, for example, my lack of self-awareness, my judgement, my fear or anxiety. What might also get in the way is my mood or my story; I need to be alert to the appropriateness of what I say, what I bring to this encounter, what I *do* with "my story".

Perhaps we have made a connection through a mutual interest we have discovered, but I need to be careful not to pursue this connection, but to hear the person's story. I might discover we have a shared interest but what is the person *really* saying? How can I curb my desire "to do" rather than "to be", to reduce the risk of focussing on what I want to do to fix this person, rather than being alongside?

**Case study**
*The patient was at first reluctant to engage with me, but as I turned to walk away a conversation started. She had leg surgery which resulted in an infection. She said angrily, "If there is a God, I can't believe that he would allow these awful things to happen to me. I have been a good person. Why does God allow that?" She talked about others who never have anything go wrong in their lives even though they are not good people. She had met two visitors previously but had declined their invitation, but she said, "You are different." She mentioned her dog, so I asked her to tell me more about him. She said that he is wonderful, but her real love and passion are her horses. Her eyes lit up, and I listened as she talked enthusiastically about them.*

## Final thoughts

Focus on the person, not the problem.

"I must listen within myself—and I must listen to what is being said to me."

## Module 4: Exploring Spirituality

"A way of naming absences and recognizing gaps..." (Swinton and Pattison 2010: 226).

In this module, we develop further the initial outline of spirituality that we provided in Module 1. Here, we offer extensive examples of descriptions and definitions of spirituality, and, throughout the session, action learning groups are invited to share and discuss which of these resonate with them as individuals and develop their understanding of the topic. As we have indicated, spiritual care is about helping the person make sense of who they are in the situation they find themselves; about encouraging their self-awareness, being able to talk about their inner life and what influences it. Spiritual care is about accompaniment in exploring a process or a search for self in relation to the world. The majority of spiritual care is to people of no faith and begins with a simple "How're you doing?" as a preliminary opening to a spiritual assessment.

In their work, Swinton and Pattison (2010) argue that, while many find spirituality hard to define, its intelligibility can grow through seeing it as individual and subjective. It is "a way of naming absences and recognizing gaps..." and so "we might use the image of putting a rope around an area of deserted land in order to allow wildlife to develop and flourish" (Swinton and Pattison 2010: 226, 234).

Swinton (2001) suggests there are five possible features of spirituality. The first is "meaning", defined as significance of life or purpose. The second is "value", which suggests cherished beliefs, truth or precious thought. Thirdly "transcendence" can be defined as appreciating "something" beyond self. The fourth feature is "connecting", meaning the relationship with self, others, environment, or possibly a sense of "otherness". The fifth feature is "becoming" meaning self-awareness, a sense of life unfolding with reflection (Swinton 2001: 25).

Pearce (2018) offers this definition: "The chaplain's listening presence *is* the pastoral encounter, with the pastoral care as the focussed listening, and the spiritual care as this space to help the storyteller to listen to themselves" (Pearce 2018: 167). Spirituality is an expression of one's inner life and journeying, in self-awareness, in deep personal needs and nourishment. Spirituality is both individual and universal, meaning everyone has it, even if unaware of it—but this is not true of religious belief. Spiritual care means "being present while the other person works it out for him or herself" (Orchard cited in Swift 2009: 175).

This lays the groundwork for introducing the idea of spiritual distress. Examples of possible causes may be trauma or crisis, bad news, a lengthy hospital stay, a life-threatening event or terminal diagnosis, a bereavement or anniversary, or a crisis connected to personal, home or work issues. The link to these examples is unexpected *change*.

Signs of spiritual distress might be tearfulness or weeping, withdrawal or lack of interest, restlessness or being unable to settle, complaining or anger. Other signs may be sudden religious leanings, or abandonment of previously held beliefs, or fear (of being alone, falling asleep, loss of control). The link here is the expression of *unarticulated emotion*.

Contrast this with religion, which may be defined as a formal or institutional set of teaching that invites belief in (a) God and a system of faith and worship which expresses an underlying spirituality. This faith is frequently interpreted in terms of particular rules, regulations, customs and practices as well as the belief content of the named religion. There is clear acknowledgement of a power other than self, usually described as "God" (Speck 2010: 91, 92).

Pastoral and spiritual care offer support to people of every faith and no faith, through respect, inclusion, dialogue, hospitality—in short, celebrating the richness of our shared humanity, regardless of the belief or values of the other person.

## Case study

*Harriet was asked to visit Henry, a retired professional once eminent in his field. His recent illness had rendered him less independent, and because of this, the relationship with his wife had broken down. Harriet wasn't sure, on the first occasion, where the conversation was going, but it was clear that Henry was both keen to talk and yet easily tired. After a series of visits, it seemed Henry was stronger and clearly looked forward to Harriet's visits. He began to talk about his spirituality, his sense of himself and where he thought these difficult circumstances were leading him. There were times when he broke down in tears. One day he said to Harriet, "How is it that I can't talk to my vicar like I can talk to you? You seem to understand what I'm going through."*

### Final thoughts

If we feel uncertain about spirituality, both in identifying it and seeing how it differs from religious belief, then perhaps if we pause and call to mind a significant event in our lives or a special moment, we will be touching our own spirituality. Feelings of profound love, or being alongside someone at a point of change in their lives, or else the mountain view or the sunset, can bring an "inner knowing" (Rohr, 2011, p. 94). These experiences touch our inner being, nourish our spirituality and they are often beyond words.

## Module 5: Dealing with Loss and Tough Conversations

> "A wounded healer is someone who can listen to a person in pain without having to speak about his or her own wounds" (Nouwen 1996: 216).

We invite participants to take a moment individually to acknowledge and reflect on their awareness or experience of grief or loss and to remember that loss, grief and bereavement may well be about things OTHER than death. What was helpful in the presence of another person who listened? What was unhelpful? If we are asked to visit someone who is experiencing some kind of loss, how do we help?

First and foremost, like in all pastoral visiting, we do not say we know how they feel or compare our experiences with theirs. We refrain from attempting to help them cheer up or divert them into something more "jolly" or even religious without listening properly. We must not avoid listening to difficult stories they may want to share. Above all, we need to avoid phrases like "God takes the best", "God is testing you" and "It's all for the best".

Grief and loss are usually about something that has changed to cause shock, loss of identity, rawness and debilitating, exhausting low mood or low self-esteem. It may reveal layers that could link with a previous hurt. We emphasize that this is a pastoral encounter, like any other, but with an even more acute awareness and sensitivity to the situation. It is important to realize that if we say, "I know how you feel..." or "Yes I've experienced grief too...", that shows the storyteller that we have lost interest in *their* story, and in *them*.

**Case study**
*John, a pastoral visitor, was asked to visit a patient called Melvyn. When he started to listen, he began to realize that Melvyn's obvious distress was not solely about being ill. As Melvyn became comfortable in talking, he revealed that his wife Celia had died about six months ago. They spoke for a while, and it was agreed that John should visit again. He listened to Melvyn talking about Celia and the good times they had, and the story developed. Melvyn missed her; he liked to think about the good times. However, it also emerged that Celia was abusive and hit Melvyn from time to time. She told him what to wear and*

*restricted his freedom. After several visits, Melvyn said to the pastoral visitor that he could not believe that someone would listen to him without judgement.*

## Tough conversations

We begin by asking the participants to take a moment to reflect on any difficult or challenging conversations: those that made them feel uncomfortable, or even annoyed them, when they did not know what to say. What about those that offended or challenged personal principles or values? What are, or could be, the barriers within ourselves that may prevent the "empty hands" and "space" needed in order to listen to others? What are the conditions that make it hard to hear? Is it that a person is saying something that conflicts with our own beliefs, values or interests? Or does it touch something in us that is uncomfortable? Might it be something that resonates with our past experience? Or perhaps, just as challenging, does it seem to make little or no sense?

As with every pastoral encounter, tough conversations demand that we create space within ourselves beforehand. In preparation for visiting, we pause and breathe. We empty our hands and put aside our own story, making space to listen to *their* story. Having taken time to do this, we are now able to commit to providing space for the person.

Tough listening can mean that first, it's tough to hear because of personal barriers, or a distressing subject, or it takes me out of my comfort zone and/or second, it's tough to hear because I'm trying to hear what's not being said, or work out *why* it's being said. Finally, it might be tough because it seems to make no rational sense, if the patient is confused for any number of reasons.

Tough issues may include someone's fixed opinion or deep-felt prejudice, or religion or belief. It might be about listening to a complaint or a distressing event. The story may include lengthy personal detail or, equally challenging, long silences. Dealing with tough issues includes listening, accepting and respecting. It means gently encouraging the person to tell their story. It also means avoiding siding with a complaint or grumbling about others. We must avoid agreeing to take responsibility to help resolve issues, and we must not collude or express a strong alternative viewpoint or offer advice.

Confidentiality is paramount. There will be occasions, however, when we feel we must ask our patient's permission to share their story if it includes active abuse, self-harm, or harm to others. Any safeguarding issues need to be communicated to the right person in authority. For hospital visitors, this of course would be a chaplain. In the case of visiting in the parish, this will be a member of the clergy. In the case of a nursing home, it should be communicated to the care home manager. Regardless of which, the information needs to be communicated carefully and sensitively.

While thinking or responding, these are important questions to ask ourselves. Why are they talking about this? Why is this important to them? Why now? Why today? We might gently ask, "What has brought this to mind? What makes you want to talk about this today, do you think?" These questions are vital tools to help encourage the patient to continue to tell their story, as they continue to work out the answers for themselves. But how do I respond when it makes no sense? Whether or not the content makes sense to us, we listen with regard for their humanity and *their* story. We must not regard "making sense" as a criterion for our decision as to whether this story is worth listening to.

**Case study**
*The patient looked at me suspiciously and then averted her eyes. Her arms were covered in scars from self-harm. She was reluctant to talk, but I remarked on a tattoo on her hand. She said, "He was taken away when he was one"; it was her son's name. She had no job but a supportive family and a boyfriend. Her previous partner had her son removed from her, and she does not see him. Normally she hides her scars with a sleeve. We talked about it being her way of coping, and she said she has had help but is not able to connect with any of the people who offer it. She is sad about not seeing her son, and she drinks and lashes out at others. We talked about music as well as her scars. She said every scar has a meaning to her.*

## Final thoughts

"Anyone who wants to pay attention without intention has to be at home in his own house—that is, he has to discover the centre of his life in his own heart" (Nouwen, 1979, p. 90).

## Module 6: Reflective Practice, Self-awareness and Self-care

"No one can be a good host who is not at home in his/her house. Nor can I be a good host until I am rooted in my own centre. Then, and only then, have I something to give others" (de Waal 2003: Chapter VII, Section 3, paragraph 1).

In this module, we aim to develop a deeper understanding of reflective practice and its place in pastoral visiting. This helps us to appreciate how this work can affect us and so this module also includes a section on how to care for oneself and work within our limits, as well as learning how to learn and develop our practice through reflection.

**Learning from experience**
How do we make sure we learn from our experiences? How can each pastoral visit help us to be a better visitor next time? This is vital to our work and development because of the essential nature of learning by reflecting on our pastoral practice (Kelly 2010: 48). Reflective practice is a key element to learning and development of good practice in pastoral and spiritual care, allowing us to explore "learning and developing through examining what we think happened ... reviewing or reliving the experience to bring it to focus" (Bolton 2010: 13). Being chaplains, we work mainly with the "intentional use of the self" (Kelly and Paterson 2013: 57). Working in the pastoral encounter requires care of ourselves as well as insight, self-awareness and the ability to see beyond the obvious or the functional.

Reflective practice skills include the "deliberate process of critically interpreting and understanding experience" (Cobb 2005: 29) and being alert to one's own "unresolved needs and conflicts" (Speck 1988: 20) but developing out of one's own woundedness (Bushell 2008: 60). What is required is "deep self-knowledge" (Swift 2009: 169) and being aware that the work means being able to "walk through ordinary doors to spend time in rooms with those whose lives have suddenly become immersed in sorrow" (Swift 2009: 169). In addition, we are to "aid people in crisis tell their own story" (Walton, H. 2002: 4), as we develop as an "empty handed" (Swift 2009: 175) and a "welcoming guest" sharing "mutual hospitality" with the visitor as "an interested guest, as a stranger in a strange land" but who equally is able "to welcome the stranger . . . to host the strange" (Walton, M. 2012: 228, 233).

## Self-care
We reiterate the challenges and demands of pastoral and spiritual care and encourage our participants to think about how they will care for themselves in order to be able to undertake this work. What do they already do to relax, be refreshed and allow themselves to be replenished?

## Exploring self-awareness
As has been explored earlier in the course, in considering how a pastoral encounter starts, the beginning is *long* before. It is vital to include in one's preparation for the visits a sense of one's own wellbeing and remember whose story we have come to the pastoral encounter to hear.

If we are to offer pastoral and spiritual care to others, we must have a sense of our own story, our needs, our personal situation and feelings and our own ability to be alongside others.

## Case study
*Jane was finding her visit with a patient quite challenging. He was a retired bishop and insisted on mentioning it several times in the conversation. He gave her a long-winded account of his ministry overseas and even supplied a monologue on what he thought pastoral and spiritual care were! Jane felt a little overwhelmed, as this was her first year as a pastoral visitor, but after a while she also found herself feeling irritated and patronized. At the end of the visit, she felt she had done little other than nod her head and listen hard. When the bishop's wife arrived by the bed, Jane felt she was all but dismissed by both patient and visitor. Back at the reflective practice session, Jane was tearful, saying she was no good at this visiting business. She unpacked her story and felt relieved that the team were willing to listen to her, share her difficult morning and encourage her to keep going. It was also helpful to ponder with the group why the bishop might have needed to recount all his achievements to her, and what that may tell us about his current situation.*

> **Final thoughts...**
>
> "Standing in the place where there are no answers, no quick exits to open, does not require the gifts of those whose hands are full. It is a situation that calls for great patience, compassion and faithfulness to the value of the human being in front of you... (which is) the product of considerable preparation, maturity and deep personal self-knowledge.
>
> For only when the chaplain's (pastoral visitor's) hands are empty will wounded people dare to offer their stories and allow their utmost shards of doubt and hope to be handled with love and honoured with insight" (Swift, 2009, p. 175).

## The "HELP" Wellbeing Reflection Tool

The HELP Wellbeing Reflection Tool is intended to guide this particular "learning from experience". The reflective cycle is an aide-memoire to prompt the discussion in the group, where each "stage" may often develop and move on seamlessly. The cycle is simply there to help.

This chapter has described the structure of our training for pastoral visitors. We now outline the way we have created opportunities to share our discoveries more widely through our collaborative conferences with regional chaplains and volunteers.

# CREATING SPACE: THE PASTORAL ENCOUNTER

## HELP Wellbeing Reflection cycle

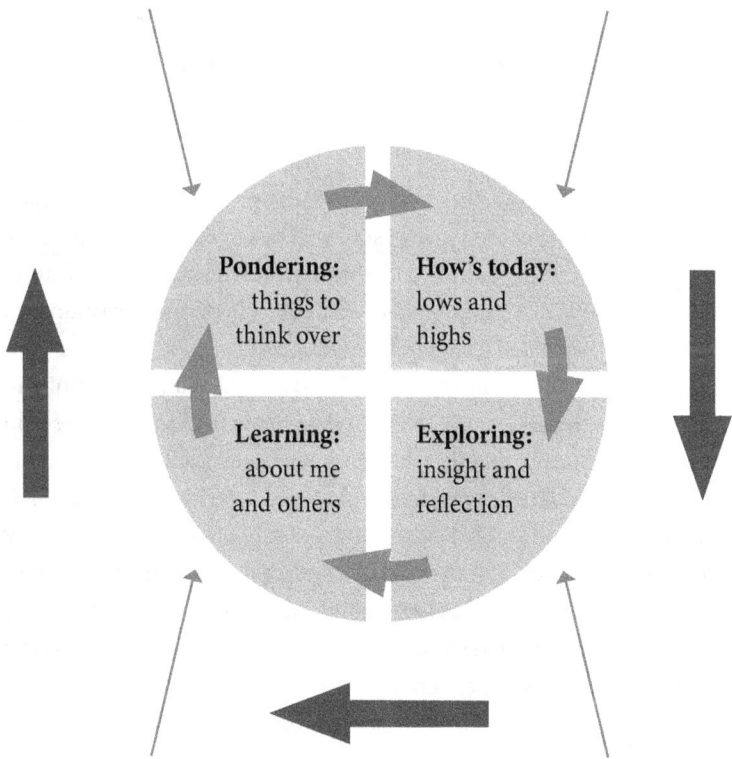

4. What do we take away from today? Things learnt? What from today will make another visit better?

1. General feelings about today's work... explore *one* really low or challenging visit & *one* fulfilling, fruitful encounter...

3. What have I learnt about how other people deal with situations? Have any of today's experiences reminded me of anything personal... to do with me... or others?

2. Explore deeper thinking—what are the deeper issues in this situation/person, this experience... or any other issues of today...

**Figure 3:** © Pearce, S. J. T., 2018, Thesis, "Building Space: Developing Reflection for Wellbeing. Can a chaplain help healthcare professionals develop reflective practice for wellbeing for themselves and their team?"

CHAPTER 6

# Conferences—teaching and nourishing a wider team

At the beginning of this story in 2009, as Sacha started his job as chaplain full-time, it had been the practice several times a year as a collaborative group of regional chaplains to gather as a means of support and sharing good practice. With a background of expanding this to include volunteers once a year, the idea of a conference developed.

The Saltash Conference (January 2010) started as an opportunity to consider how to use our volunteers in chaplaincy research with the help of Dr Harriet Mowat, following her 2008 published chaplaincy audit. The audit recommendations encouraged chaplains to be involved in research in order to generate a more evidenced-based support for their developing professional practice. One of our colleagues was embarking on a Master's degree and was exploring the use of our department, analysing the means of recording pastoral and spiritual encounters with patients, which later became a chapter in a chaplaincy textbook (Baxendale 2015).

In Saltash, within the first few minutes of the conference, it was clear that the volunteers present had little or no awareness of being part of something like this. With seamless skill, Dr Mowat divided the volunteer attendees into mixed groups and invited them to talk together about their bedside visits, to discuss what they thought went on during them and to share their experiences. Sacha facilitated one particular group, many of whom were from other hospitals. He describes this as something that just happened naturally, instinctively helping them reflect on their time as pastoral visitors and encouraging them to look back at any particular visit that stood out for them in the recent past. It was very clear that, while many had not had this opportunity before, several of them were so very much in need of sharing their story. At least a couple of them later expressed their gratitude for having the space to talk. Towards the end of this session, Dr Mowat came to observe and later discussed with Sacha that this practice of the chaplain helping pastoral visitor volunteers to reflect may be a practice for him to research.

The following year Bishop Martin Shaw led the conference and invited consideration of what a pastoral visitor actually does as they visit patients. In essence, he was encouraging them to recognize their contribution to the pastoral encounter as more than just a social visit. His delightful sense of humour and direct style were intended to inspire them to actually enjoy what they were doing. This was indeed new ground for those for whom bedside visiting was another example of "doing good works"! For many this conference was unsettling, but for others it was both comforting and constructive.

By 2012, Sacha had begun the first stage of his doctoral study and co-hosted the conference in Plymouth with another colleague as they shared early discoveries about the way in which the department was developing. For two years, the team had been making early steps in reflecting together and also in growing more aware of a rather broader understanding of spirituality. Totally unrehearsed, Sacha asked the Plymouth volunteers who were attending what they felt about using the new reflective practice in their meeting at the end of their morning visits, instead of undertaking a detailed handover of their visits. Two of them replied with energy and enthusiasm, saying what a difference it made and how much they were learning from one another. Indeed, they generously said how proud they were to be part of the team! This was very encouraging, combined with inviting people to look more closely at the work they were doing, in terms of exploring how to define pastoral and spiritual care. We were keen to continue to contribute to the annual conference!

Sharing the hosting once more in 2013, this time with a chaplain from a different hospital, Sacha offered more of the developments that were emerging in our own pastoral training course. The conference was entitled "Staying when it's tough—leaving when it's time", which explored the timing of the pastoral encounter and then the self-care afterwards. The first session invited people firstly to reflect on their experiences of visiting and then listening skills: how to be alongside someone and truly listen with gentleness and patience, to be alert and a willing hearer. As was described more fully in Chapter 1, the image of having "empty hands" (Swift 2009: 175) in order to hold someone else's story was introduced. They also explored coping with stories that are difficult to hear and the role of silence. The volunteers were invited to reflect on what they wanted to achieve in their visiting and how to make best use of their visiting time. They were also introduced to the pastoral encounter as agenda-free, "being present while the other person works it out for him or herself" (Orchard cited in Swift 2009: 175) and the "welcoming guest" of "mutual hospitality" (Walton, M. 2012: 226) image as their role.

In 2013, the middle session of the day, led by the other co-host, offered brief reflections on the Francis Report that had just been published, inviting healthcare professionals to be more caring and compassionate. Attendees were asked to consider its significance.

For the final session, Sacha explored further awareness of reflective practice in terms of using it as a tool to make the most out of a pastoral visit and to allow each patient encounter to help us become a better visitor next time. Participants also looked at historical evidence for reflective practice being a means of learning from experience, drawing on familiar names such as fifth-century BC Confucius and Plato. There was also exploration of reflection during a visit as "reflection-in-action" (Schön 1983) and "living human documents" (Graham 2009: 151) as the image of themselves being a source of their own learning. Further encouraged to let the pastoral visit help learning, they were invited to see its value because "pastoral practice not reflected upon is practice that only partially fulfils its potential" (Kelly 2010: 48). The closing plenary was called "Ready Once More".

For the following three years, colleagues across the region shared between them the responsibility for the annual conferences and they followed particular chaplaincy-related topics such as bereavement, dementia, end-of-life and mental health subjects. Although clearly these are important issues, we reflected that the conference should have a more "sharing of resources" purpose, gathering pastoral care volunteers from several different contexts. This provides the opportunity to learn from one another and not necessarily always involve outside resources. We offered to take the responsibility for the 2017 conference once more.

## "Creating Space: The Pastoral Encounter" (2017)

After several years of conferences that presented a particular theme, we decided that the focus of the next conference would be a return to the actual dynamics of the pastoral encounter. What is going on as we visit? How do we best prepare ourselves for this work and what is it that we are really offering the patient? Setting apart the value of conferences that have a specialist theme, how can we share the essence or anatomy of a patient visit?

The emphasis here was on our shared discoveries. What actually has worked for us and what have we found that is worth sharing across teams? What place does reflective practice have in our volunteer team and what does it look like in action?

Our aim was to present the main points of our training course, an updated version of which has already been described in Chapter 5. We began by outlining our definitions of pastoral, spiritual and religious care before any other teaching material was covered and then we proceeded to emphasize the notion of "creating space" to share the idea that pastoral volunteers and chaplains were not visiting to "deliver" something, but to create space for the patient.

We also spoke about the dangers of expectations for both patient and visitor and especially the assumption that a patient would automatically want any kind of religious care. In some traditional chaplaincy volunteer teams, the questioning of this assumption is not always well received. We have been aware of team members from other hospitals who distribute various religious symbols, one might say indiscriminately, during patient visits and teams that are more focussed on religion than others.

Our experience has been that such teams expect a conference day to begin with prayers and to have a more religious (usually Christian) theme, so it is worth saying that whilst we subsequently received much appreciation through feedback of this day, a small number of delegates were disappointed that we held a period of silence at the start of the day rather than prayers, and they reported that we did not mention God enough for them. We had anticipated this and indeed, our anticipation was the reason why we had chosen to use this conference opportunity to explore the basics of what chaplaincy is about and how that is reflected in pastoral visiting.

We used the collection of patient and visitor feedback via the "whiteboard" (see Chapter 4) to show that visiting without an agenda and with empty hands has a wealth of data in the form of quotes to support its effectiveness, for example:

> "When you said, 'We don't talk about religion,' the patient sighed with relief."

> "I really enjoyed talking to you, because you didn't say anything!"

> "You were the right person at the right time."

> "I was all right pretending until you came along!"

This was an opportunity to encourage other chaplaincy teams to try out their own version of the whiteboard as a means of capturing data on the patient's perception of pastoral visiting, which in turn helps the team to grow and evolve to meet patient need more appropriately.

Our final session of the day was a live demonstration of a reflective practice group using members of our own team. This regular opportunity is not available to all chaplaincy departments and so it seemed like the ideal moment for all delegates to see a session in action. Four volunteers and two chaplains sat in a semicircle at the front of the room. Prior to this, the group had been asked to imagine a visit they had conducted recently in readiness to discuss it at this session and to change or omit any distinguishing features of the patient story to preserve confidentiality. One chaplain facilitated the session and the other shared a story of a visit too. Many delegates reported afterwards that they had found this demonstration significantly more helpful than a verbal description of how reflective practice worked.

Our keynote speaker at this 2017 conference was Dame Bishop Sarah Mullally, the then Bishop of Crediton and now Bishop of London. It was a great honour to have Bishop Sarah commend the day's teaching and to encourage chaplains and volunteers alike in their vital work.

## "Creating Space for me" (planned for 2022)

Sometimes we forget, and new volunteers might not be aware, that the work of pastoral and spiritual care is demanding and not simply a cosy chat to cheer someone up. If we are doing it right, it takes energy and makes demands on us; therefore we need to look after ourselves. This conference focusses on self-care, reminding us again that a powerful image of chaplaincy is our "empty hands": "For only when the chaplain's hands are empty will wounded people dare to offer their stories and allow their most intimate shards of doubt and hope to be handled with love and honoured with insight" (Swift 2009: 175). This means being sufficiently able to put aside one's own story, making space to listen, becoming the "empty hands" for them to fill with their story. If one is burdened with one's own issues, one cannot give honour and full attention to the other, and is unable to listen properly, with insufficient emotional intelligence not to be overwhelmed by the challenge of what is being said. In order to reflectively "empty my hands", I must first consider the question, "But what am I carrying?"

## Silent space

We begin by offering ten minutes of silence, with rolling images on a screen that encourage a stilling of the self. Delegates can choose to pray or meditate or do nothing during this period. Offering the choice of how to use the ten minutes is a reflection of the day's theme: that each of us will find a means of caring for ourselves that will most likely vary. For those who have previously expected to have prayer at the start of a conference, the space to just do that is available. For those who want to simply be still, the same space easily provides that. Even before any formal input to the conference, we are therefore acknowledging a need and a provision for preparation in a gentle, silent space that all may use. In past conferences, the majority of delegates have expressed their deep appreciation for this silent space. A small number have expressed disappointment that we do not specifically invite vocal prayer, so by offering this silent space we give the opportunity for everyone to take ownership for what will help them prepare for the learning ahead and use the silent space accordingly.

## My Space—self-care and "being" not "doing"

The first session begins by revisiting the concept outlined in Chapter 1 of being "empty handed" (Swift 2009: 175) as a prerequisite to creating space for the patient to tell their story; it looks at why this concept is critical, and how we place an emphasis on our presence constituting "being" and not "doing". This in turn leads to the question of "what am I carrying?", not just on a particular morning but as a long-term story or set of stories pertinent to one's life. We encourage delegates to think about how they create space for themselves before visiting, to be self-aware about the stories, both short- and long-term, that they carry, and to look at how they manage to hold or set aside their narrative to avoid interrupting a patient story. This setting aside of our stories may be hard work in its own right. Our skilled volunteers have told us that this setting aside creates its own exhaustion. They and we are not simply sitting on our hands to stop ourselves doing something practical; we are holding our own stories in the background, so they do not intrude on a pastoral visit, and in its own right this "holding" demands additional energy and effort. In action learning groups, we encourage volunteers to talk about times they have had to put aside their own stories and, in a subsequent plenary, to share some of these examples in the wider conference audience.

Not only is this setting the scene for a conference on self-care, it is also a formal acknowledgement that this work is demanding; it is not simply visiting the sick with a light-hearted cheeriness. Pastoral and spiritual care is about a willingness to offer space and to not let our own stories invade that space. In the light of this, we ask ourselves, "What is it that sustains us?" and we acknowledge that self-care is vital if we are to undertake this work well. In action learning groups, we share our stories of what we do to take care of ourselves, if we have already discovered this.

## Creating "my space" workshops

Delegates are offered the opportunity to sample a maximum of two short workshops lasting thirty minutes, which run twice during the afternoon. The workshops planned are poetry, origami, meditation and craft. They should be conducted in a quiet environment and even if the workshop necessitates speaking (for example the poetry workshop) it should be nevertheless conducted with space for quiet reflection alongside speaking.

## Reflecting on "Creating my Space"

The workshops are followed by a plenary where delegates are encouraged to share the experience of their day, including the workshops, within the context of a reflective practice cycle. How was it? What did you learn? What will you take away from this day? Is it a new idea for you that pastoral visiting demands self-care? How will you care for yourself more than you do already?

Thus far, we have provided a story of our developing use of regional chaplaincy conferences to share our discoveries more widely: our teaching, our learning and our encouragement, alongside chaplains and pastoral visitors from other hospital trusts.

We have shown how our contribution has developed over more than ten years. This includes our increasing focus on both developing people's awareness of the real experience of the pastoral encounter and learning from it. Our contribution also develops awareness of the vital nature of self-care in this work for all in the chaplaincy team. This part of our story is an entry into a wider realm of sharing our discoveries.

We will now explore the ways in which our discoveries have been developed within the hospital context, and, moving beyond the hospital building, how they have been shared in local parishes and dioceses.

CHAPTER 7

# Sharing "learning from discoveries"

This part of our story takes us to new discoveries both within the hospital context and, over time, to different places and people. Here we first outline the way in which our pastoral training course has developed over the years or, more particularly, its methodology, the steps of its evolution. We then describe the part of the journey where we have gone beyond the hospital walls into parish communities, clergy and lay minister gatherings, as well as involving a number of different groups as our trainees. We also explore the way in which, as a result of these several developments, how the actual pastoral training material has evolved and continues to do so. Sharing our learning from discoveries takes healthcare chaplaincy out of the hospital context to a wider constituency but also means that the whole diversity of people and places share new learning and discoveries together. This, we argue, shows our story as a model of both practical and public theology.

At this point, it is helpful to note that there are two parallel stories or journeys here. One of them describes the developments within the hospital context and the other, which sometimes runs contemporaneously, is our growing relationship and discoveries with people from other places. The latter may be either trainees to whom we have delivered the course, physically in their context, or those who have come into the hospital be trained with us within our building. Once again, each story or journey helps the other, each learning in a profoundly symbiotic way. This mirrors our experience of the chaplain in the pastoral encounter (see Chapter 1) of the "mutual hospitality" (Walton, M. 2012: 226) of both those involved, which creates space that turns "blurred encounters to thresholds of transformation" (Reader and Baker 2009: 219). This means that reflecting on two stories creates space for and develops something wholly new for both of them.

## Hospital context: developing the course, the venue and the candidates (2010–16)

The venue for training pastoral visitor volunteers in the hospital has always been something of a challenge in terms of finding and booking an appropriate and large enough meeting room. Over a number of years we regularly discussed but resisted using the multi-faith prayer room or the chapel and, on several occasions, tried to shoehorn three chaplains and twelve trainee volunteers into one of our larger offices to an almost claustrophobic effect!

There came a time in around 2013 to 2014 when, having started to make use of a good-sized training room elsewhere on the hospital site, we reflected that having groups any larger than twelve meant that we were unable to observe how our trainees were developing. We had inherited a rather didactic style of course material in 2009/2010 (imagine Ronnie Corbett telling a story from an armchair!) which was totally focussed on delivery rather than helpful observation or discernment of candidates. There were a number of courses where several trainees, who had already been involved in their own pastoral church work, left and did not engage with us post-course, leaving without starting their volunteering in the hospital. There were also those who really showed little aptitude for pastoral care work. We needed to revise our teaching style and group size. During this period, we were slowly moving from delivering solely by reading from home-grown handouts to using both the printed material and visual screen presentations. However, we were losing more volunteers than we were gaining.

Prior to running a training course, the department had always interviewed potential pastoral visitors, sought references and required both health and safeguarding checks. However, the interview, albeit very informal, was done by a single chaplain one-to-one with the candidate. Eventually, by 2016, we had decided to interview with two chaplains and made clearer to the potential volunteer that this would be a means of all three of us taking time to discern whether our work was the right place for them, and indeed whether they were the right people for us.

The course itself had been run annually, but from 2012 we were delivering it twice a year in spring and autumn. There were seven three-hour sessions, one per week, for a whole afternoon. The candidates all came from a faith background, mostly Christian, although in the early years of this story we had a Muslim member of staff volunteering and in subsequent years have valued, at different times, three Buddhist volunteers. Recruitment was initially done by writing to local churches. We puzzled how we should advertise to a wider audience for a broader field of candidates. Advertising with a local volunteer agency in 2012 proved helpful, as did the local University of the Third Age. Interestingly today our recruitment is mostly by word of mouth.

At the end of each course, we took time to review and revise our material. Beyond the handbook and the PowerPoint, a new chaplain, who was obliged to do the course at the start of their post in 2016, suggested we use case studies. This of course was the right idea and remains a key element of our training today. However, at the time we had so much material and in each training session we were often pushed for time, with the twenty-one-hour course exhausting for everyone. Revisions had to continue.

Combined with a change of focus on recruiting and the desire to continue to adjust this from a faith-focussed course to have an increasingly greater emphasis on spirituality and reflection, we wondered more about delivering the course elsewhere. By beginning to edit out the material that was hospital-specific, it was possible to share it in 2013 with a parish group. Back in the hospital, we were also approached in 2016 by a local lay chaplain, who was then involved in providing pastoral care volunteers for local care homes, and since then we have welcomed a number of similar external trainees to the course. Again, modifications were made as the trainee group in the hospital came now from two differing contexts, some to remain with us as pastoral visitor volunteers on the wards and others to return to volunteer in local care homes. Already the benefit of diversity was beginning to show.

## Parish context: sharing discoveries (2013)

Meanwhile, sharing chaplaincy with people from other contexts, initially with parish groups, began in 2013 in a parish local to Sacha when he was invited to teach their pastoral visitor team. Some of their existing pastoral team had received local diocesan training in the past while several new people were joining with some experience but no training. The expectation was that post-training, they would be given regular ongoing support from the new incumbent in due course. In consultation with their lay ministers and then the new incumbent, they received a seven-week course, in two-hour sessions one evening a week, using material from our pastoral care course that we were using at the time. The venue was in the home of one of the trainees, taking over their dining room with computer, data projector and large screen, and supper plus one chaplain and eight volunteers!

With slight modifications, and removing the hospital-specific content, this was the first attempt at adapting material that was being used in the hospital context for use in the parish setting. This was very well received at the time and is still mentioned in local church circles, although there has been no opportunity to follow up or update the volunteers, who essentially manage their own visiting informally. Currently one of the attendees of the 2013 training course co-ordinates a much smaller team and liaises with the current incumbent.

## Hospital context: sharing discoveries with the Church diocese (2017)

As keynote speaker at our 2017 chaplaincy conference (described in Chapter 6), Bishop Sarah witnessed significant elements of the pastoral and spiritual care discoveries we were sharing, including our profound belief in the use of reflective practice. With her background, prior to ordination, in a highly successful nursing career and now as a senior leader in the Church, we felt very affirmed by her support and her invitation to consider sharing our training material with the diocese. We were encouraged to suggest to them that pastoral training may best come from those who work routinely in the context of the hospital environment, meaning always in the face of acute human need. This affirmed our sense that healthcare chaplaincy had something to offer and our desire to share our discoveries with the wider Church. In due course, we were approached by the diocesan secretary inviting us to report even more widely on our "learning from discoveries" by taking part in a presentation entitled "Models of Chaplaincy" within the Exeter Diocesan Synod. Using this opportunity to speak to a clergy audience, mostly from a parish setting or outlook, we were able to highlight how our ethos has evolved from providing what is assumed to be largely religious care to a much wider remit of "being alongside" and creating space for anything the patient wishes to discuss. Hence we shared the ideas that pastoral encounter is a valuable source of learning. We validate our practice with reflection and learning through peer review and "what the patient thinks". It provides another angle on the adventure of learning and journeying together.

We reiterated our current definitions of pastoral, spiritual and religious care to root our presentation in the context in which we find ourselves working and how our discoveries shape our continued work and our training. Again, we described how the qualitative data that we collect and report via our whiteboard (see Chapter 4) is used to continually shape our way of working and how it provides a way of "checking out" what the patient really thinks of our pastoral care from the point of view of being a recipient, or better, in a shared partnership with us. Several of the quotes from the whiteboard, by now familiar to the reader, were shared:

"I really enjoyed talking to you because you didn't say anything!"

"You stayed and we talked about everyday things."

"When I said, 'We don't talk about religion', the patient sighed with relief."

"You listening to my story is such a release."

There are many more available quotes in our repertoire, but these are a selection of the examples that powerfully reflect how attentive listening with no accompanying agenda appears to be highly valued by the patient. Diocesan Synod expressed appreciation of our presentation, and interest in our newly formed ideas about how we might share this training with parishes, and other communities, who might benefit from a wider canvas when training for pastoral care provision.

## Parish context: sharing discoveries (2018)

Following the interest expressed at Diocesan Synod, we tailored our course to a request from one of Jan's local parish teams to teach "Creating Space" to their pastoral visitors. As a first step, the rector of the parish was willing to host a pilot scheme for this, first inviting current and would-be Eucharistic ministers to the course. In fact, another local church of a different denomination sent an additional two of its pastoral visitors to join in, making this a group of nine trainees.

Developing from the experience of teaching in a parish in 2013, we reflected that this would probably once again involve gathering in the early evening and that, with careful editing and condensing of the material, it would be possible to run six sessions of two hours. Once again, as we had begun to find in the hospital-based training, even a small element of diversity in the trainees' context proved fruitful in terms of shared stories and learning together from among themselves and not only from our training material.

The outcome was very encouraging, and we were not surprised to hear that this teaching had been well received. Feedback was thus:

> "Absolutely recommend! It gave me valuable insight in drawing closer to others in a deeper, more meaningful way."

> "The course has helped me in developing a closer listening ear to everyone I encounter."

"Stimulating, encouraging, thought-provoking and personally fulfilling."

"I have really enjoyed this course. It has helped me to reflect on previous skills/experiences and apply them to a pastoral setting. I am going to miss our evenings! Thank you so much."

## Hospital venue, mixed context: learning together in action learning groups (2019)

Drawing together the parish and diocesan experience, by 2017 we had trained people as pastoral visitors for three different contexts: hospital, care homes and the parish community. It was clear from our parish training feedback and encouragement from Diocesan Synod that "Creating Space" as a training course could reach well beyond the limits of preparing volunteers for hospital-based pastoral visiting. The scope of the training was highly relevant and there was interest in its provision for wider groups. However, the problem lay in the logistics of delivery, since Devon is a large county and the three course trainers were already mostly full-time chaplains. The evening pilot scheme in the second parish setting, although receiving successful acknowledgement, confirmed our suspicions that we would not be able to deliver this training parish by parish and continue to undertake our day jobs as chaplains too. It was thanks to one of our non-teaching colleagues, who suggested we attempt to train both hospital and non-hospital visitors alongside one another in a single location, that a new incarnation of the course was born. During the course of writing this chapter in early pandemic lockdown, we could never have imagined the idea of delivering the course remotely to obviate these difficulties. We return to this proposition in Chapter 10.

The next course, held in autumn 2018, was run in our hospital at the end of a working day, and as the applications increased, both internally and externally, from this point we finally decided to use the chapel as a training venue. Again, we ran six two-hour sessions, as we had done in the parish.

By 2019 and into 2020, we had received interest from several current pastoral visitors from parishes and three undergraduates studying counselling and psychotherapy, who had applied to us for a short-term placement in the hospital. We also had curates on placement, volunteers from other parts of the hospital, clergy and laity from churches, volunteers from care homes and of course several expressing interest in becoming our "own" potential hospital visitors! The course content continued to assume a more generic and widely applicable remit, with all hospital-specific teaching material being taught subsequently to hospital pastoral visitors as they began their ward visiting with us.

From our experience at the 2017 chaplaincy conference, as described in the previous chapter, we considered, with now increasingly large numbers of trainees, how to further develop the benefit of diversity in the trainees' context. We reflected also from the much earlier experience of how to avoid the mistakes of not noticing how they were progressing or developing through the course. At the 2017 conference, we had made a table plan for the one hundred-plus attending in order to separate hospital teams; this was to encourage people from differing contexts to share their stories and listen to each other, to help reflection and shared learning. For the spring course in 2019, we applied the same principle and saw once again the value of people from differing contexts, and yet with the same purpose, reflecting together. This use of "action learning groups" gave the opportunity to teach and learn together through each course session. It was both interesting and energizing to see each trainee allocated a group to which they would belong for the duration of the course which would provide a focus for reflecting together at each point in the training where group discussion was appropriate. Most importantly the groups were deliberately mixed so that those in each group were from a different source (potential hospital visitor, parish visitor, student) so they could offer differing viewpoints on the discussion each time, whatever the learning topic.

In Chapter 5, we discussed how the course had evolved to teach reflective practice from Week 1, so that candidates could use this skill from the very beginning of the course to reflect on all that was being taught week by week. With the addition of action learning groups, we were able not only to teach reflective practice, but to enable the actual practice to take place in groups during the training sessions themselves, as well as the expected self-reflection on course material that we encouraged between weekly sessions.

In addition, the advantage of varied group membership was that the teaching material could be discussed from the different contexts that individual group members were to find themselves in as pastoral visitors. The variation in trainee "home" contexts when they were encouraged to participate in whole-audience discussion meant that the trainee input into a session influenced the teaching material not only in a very fruitful way, but in a way that departed significantly from the input that might have been witnessed in the early days of the course, when it was taught largely to volunteers who were mostly from church backgrounds. Young undergraduates undertaking sociology or counselling and psychotherapy degrees have differing life experiences and learning from which to contribute, as do those non-hospital trainees who have home visiting skills, or latterly, clergy who have attended recent training with us, who offer a different perspective again.

It appears that in trying to solve the logistical problem of course delivery we have stumbled upon a new and much more effective way of teaching "Creating Space" to a variety of trainees, who contribute to the course in novel and varied ways, and we have now adopted the shape of training in action learning groups for all future courses. An additional advantage of opening out our training to differing groups is that we are in a more beneficial position to attract new applicants and reach new contexts. Recently, we have been invited to a local university to talk to undergraduates about hospital-based placements for pastoral visiting and the response has been very enthusiastic. By providing training to these placement students prior to their work with us, we are doing all we can to ensure they are well prepared for hospital visiting, but we are also offering them valuable experience and training which will contribute to their future work opportunities.

## Reflecting on sharing learning from discoveries

As we have argued so far, *Creating Space* is a story of the "being" of healthcare chaplaincy and a story of an ongoing energy to learn. By sharing, and continuing to share with others our practical theology, our contextual dialogue of narrative and praxis (Graham 2005, 2012), we demonstrate that our story and learning are synergetic with those among whom we work at every level. Whether we are listening to a patient's story and empowering them to hear it for themselves, or whether we are reflecting with healthcare staff or our team, or facilitating a pastoral session, each is an encounter of being and learning for each involved.

While showing *our* context of healthcare chaplaincy as a paradigm of practical theology, we also demonstrate public theology in our context, with "chaplaincy in the public square" (Todd 2011) and a ministry as "chaplain standing in the world... and looking around" (Walters 2017: 51). As has also been outlined in Chapter 1, here theology is a way of thinking, where for chaplains "theology is their expertise" and as "a source of nurture, challenge and insight" (Pattison 2015b: 111, 126) with religion as an example and not an end in itself. Our practice invites the insights of faith to provide the language of transformation and change, journeying and discovery. It is a source of new life revealed in the public place. We are not in the business of active proselytizing, but our work is by our presence "standing alongside individuals and institutions to nurture citizenship and human flourishing", to "seek and promote justice for the disenfranchised" with "enacted parables of care and witness" as their "creative endeavour" (Pattison 2015b: 126). We show this not only at the interface between chaplain and patients, visitors and healthcare staff, but also chaplain and pastoral visitor volunteer and all the numbers of people from a variety of other contexts within and outside the hospital, within and outside the Church.

Having demonstrated this in this chapter with the story of sharing our learning from discoveries, we will now, in a different way, explore the identity of the chaplain, as we share our experiences of "finding a chaplain".

CHAPTER 8

# Finding a chaplain: discernment— what does a chaplain look like?

Our story of healthcare chaplaincy shares our discoveries both within the hospital context and well beyond, as *our* contextual dialogue of narrative and praxis (Graham 2005, 2012). As we have shown, this includes nurturing and being alongside those involved in pastoral care in the face of the whole miasma of human experiences. We have shown and argue that our story provides a refreshing model towards developing the practical and public theology of the life of the Church. Here we shall describe our experiences of working alongside both laity and clergy, accompanying them on their journey of discernment. We shall show how this informs our claim that the unique ministry of healthcare chaplaincy must now in the twenty-first century be acknowledged and celebrated as a well-defined, discernible vocation alongside, but neither dominated by nor dependent on, the "one-size-fits-all" traditional parish model of ordained ministry.

## Curates on chaplaincy placement

Jan's own initial experience of acute hospital chaplaincy consisted of one morning a week visiting patients and sharing reflective practice at the end of the morning with chaplains and volunteers.

From Jan's perspective on chaplaincy placements, the most obvious observation is that being exposed to this novel environment with its different challenges and then reflecting on one's reaction to the experience will be an important—albeit initial—litmus test of whether this is the right place to be. In other words, this environment has to excite as well as challenge and perhaps even terrify the potential chaplain. Despite fears of inadequacy and monumental quantities of things to learn, it felt it was the right place for Jan to be in ministry. Paradoxically, there was a strong sense of feeling at home despite this being a completely new environment, and she could only assume this was an indication that whilst there was a great deal to learn, there was also something she could offer, which might be her background in therapy and counselling and experience with group reflection. But she also wants to emphasize that this sense of "fit" is not simply about skills and abilities—the "doing". It is also about a sense of fit from a "being" point of view. Is this person someone who can "do a chaplain's job" or are they a chaplain deep within themselves? From Jan's subsequent position in full-time chaplain employment, she observed this effect in curates who undertook placements with us. For most, but not all, there was a sense of feeling "this is where I should be". As a selection criterion, that sounds worryingly subjective, but if this "sense of fit" is accurate, there is an accompanying sense in the observing, experienced team chaplains that this placement person "looks at home, looks right" in this role. In colloquial terms, we find ourselves saying "they get it"—meaning they appear to have the temperament, the sensitivity and the personal skills, even in embryo. We can assess the potential of a chaplain by using one (but not the only) essential criterion that is also a good predictor of an effective and compassionate pastoral volunteer, and that is the willingness to be open and to learn. This is just as important as existing skills or qualifications. We have been less enthused by both pastoral volunteers and clergy placements who decide they already know what it takes to be a visitor or chaplain and are unwilling to consider trying out a new perspective.

From my subsequent position in full-time chaplain employment, I observed this effect in curates who undertook placements with us. For most, but not all, there was a sense of feeling "this is where I should be". As a selection criterion, that sounds worryingly subjective, but if this "sense of fit" is accurate, there is an accompanying sense in the observing, experienced team chaplains that this placement person "looks at home, looks right" in this role. In colloquial terms, we find ourselves saying "they get it"—meaning they appear to have the temperament, the sensitivity and the personal skills, even in embryo. We can assess the potential of a chaplain by using one (but not the only) essential criterion that is also a good predictor of an effective and compassionate pastoral volunteer, and that is *the willingness to be open and to learn*. This is just as important as existing skills or qualifications. We have been less enthused by both pastoral volunteers and clergy placements who decide they already know what it takes to be a visitor or chaplain and are unwilling to consider trying out a new perspective.

Placement therefore has an important role to play in discernment. It is an opportunity to experience the work that is pertinent to chaplaincy, not simply as an objective description and understanding of chaplaincy, but as a chance for the individual to reflect on whether or not this work "feels right" for them. It is also a chance for experienced chaplains to assess the skills and character of the individual on placement and their potential to become a chaplain, should they desire to pursue this route.

## Parish clergy and study days

Empowering others and being alongside those discerning their future is a key element of chaplaincy whether the other person is a patient, member of staff or visitor. This is also true of our support of clergy and developing a greater understanding today in people's awareness of the true ministry of the chaplain. Early in the *Creating Space* story, from 2011, there have been clergy study days run by Sacha with the support of both fellow chaplains and experienced pastoral visitors. His early study of practical theology from 2010 provided a link with a suggestion from diocesan vocational sources that curates may value some guidance on "hospital visiting" as a study day or session. This developed for several years in various forms as a session on the diocesan clergy ministerial development calendar. The first of these in May 2011 aimed to explore the reality of healthcare ministry; to aid reflection on one's own pastoral and spiritual care, in the parish or elsewhere; and to offer a fresh understanding of our shared ministries in the light of today's study of practical theology.

The full study day combined an opportunity for the visiting clergy to shadow a chaplain out on to the wards to explore the pastoral and spiritual encounter. They were invited to consider how this hospital experience related to, or may even refresh, aspects of their parish ministry. They were then involved in a reflective session to see how reflective practice was beginning to be used to learn from the morning's visits. The afternoon sessions explored the "craft" (Bushell 2008: 60) of the chaplain, with the definitions of pastoral and spiritual care being developed and the chance to consider the differences between parish and chaplaincy ministry. This included whether in chaplaincy there were differences between working generically or denominationally. The second afternoon session explored defining practical theology and considering both the theological and moral dilemmas, including issues such as the chaplain being the patient's advocate and the hospital's conscience. The session moved on to consider the theology and challenge of the occasional offices in the acute care environment, including tools for liturgy such as emergency baptisms and marriages, end-of-life care, death and bereavement. Naturally the day concluded with plenary reflections on the experiences of the day.

This study day was very well received and ran as a full day on three occasions over two years (2011, 2012). In order to help parish clergy to find diary time for this study, it became a shorter half-day, focussing on pastoral visiting, reflection on the chaplain's role and the difference between spiritual and religious care. The half-day also included reflections on the difference in terms of focus and expectation if one visits the hospital as local clergy or as the chaplain. These half-days have run annually for five years (2012, 2013, 2014, 2018 and 2019). These study days, involving experience and reflection opportunities, have thrown light on the discernment path for several clergy who over time have become chaplain colleagues in one way or another.

## Curates on placement: two-way discerning

Following the realization of the right "fit" of Jan's "coming home" to healthcare chaplaincy, completing her curacy and then joining the team full-time in 2013, we have had the privilege of creating space for several other curates to explore and discern their future ministry. They have come from differing backgrounds, but at a point in their curacy when they are ready to consider the next step. Some have attended one of our study days, for new clergy to experience hospital visiting, or else chosen to work in either a short or long placement with us. Some have come thinking that they may want to combine parish and chaplaincy ministry, while others have felt a strong call to an ordained vocation that meets people at the interface of their acute human experiences. The consistent theme is their sense that there is a ministry for them that does not necessarily solely follow the parish model but is closer to the pastoral non-agenda ministry to which they feel called.

A colleague a number of years ago spoke of there being two ways to discern a chaplain: either noticing someone who was born to it, an intuitive chaplain, or else noticing someone who is open to it and can learn it. We have certainly seen both but, as has been said, the most important feature is discerning someone's "being". This has been outlined in Chapter 1 in terms of identifying someone open for a unique model of ministry, a very particular presence, in an uncertain and changing place, of a particular kind of person.

In essence the "fit", the person being a chaplain within themselves, is often visible very early on. The volunteer, or ordinand, deacon or priest, who may have a vocation to healthcare chaplaincy, is someone who sees "the centre on the edge" (Guite 2012: 15). While totally respecting and wishing to work within the authority of the Church, they nevertheless sense a call into the remote, lying beyond or no-man's-land of a public ministry, in the "hinterland" or "wilderness" (Moody 1999: 15), meaning an accompanying ministry that "meets people where they are" (Mowat and Swinton 2007: 30), regardless of where that is, as the priority. This is being a "chaplain standing in the world... and looking around" (Walters 2017: 51). There is quickly an affirmation that this person has no agenda, save for the wellbeing of the other in the pastoral encounter, by their immediate grasping of our understanding of the difference between spiritual and religious care, their total desire to empower the other person to seek his/her own deepening, longer lasting and more strengthening self-awareness, solace and solution. However, those who offer a hint of merely being willing to pay lip-service to working in this "insecure and uncertain landscape" (Swift 2009: 122) but would feel more secure in reaching first for even unsought religious care as their priority, will probably find a ministry elsewhere. A chaplain is not someone who brings

God to the bedside, but knows God is already there, even if unbidden or undesired, and leaves God to decide how, when and in what way God may wish to be revealed.

Quite simply, we have found the very best "fit" of chaplain is someone who has a passion for pastoral care as a ministry of listening and prompting the storyteller; for spiritual care as a ministry of being alongside, helping the other hear their own story in the telling of it and in their own reflections; and for religious care, offering it only if it is sought. In many situations, this discernment is easily revealed, although it can take the Church a while to endorse the otherwise glaringly obvious gift, passion and pastoral heart.

## Pastoral visitor volunteer to chaplain: A courageous journey

This is Pat's story of her journey from experienced pastoral visitor to ordinand, in training to be a deacon, and who, while in training, became an honorary chaplain, and thence was employed part-time in a job-share role as palliative and oncology chaplain.

Pat trained as pastoral visitor with us in 2010. Her volunteer work grew over time to be for three days a week, and she provided highly motivated, outstanding quality and wide-ranging pastoral and spiritual care with increasing responsibility. Her significant and evolving pastoral and spiritual care skills meant that our deep sense of her increasing calling in this role grew, which led us towards further developing in this specialist ministry as an exceptionally gifted lay chaplain. Our sense was to seek authorization for what she was already doing *and* supporting her in further development by exploring her calling as a distinctive deacon based as an honorary chaplain here in healthcare.

We had absolutely no reservation in warmly recommending her for further discernment of the development of her chaplaincy vocation. Despite our first approach to the diocese in 2015, there were apparently some doubts from an academic and, in part, parish perspective. However, from the diocesan vocational support, she was encouraged to explore her lay ministry in pastoral care as her place of ongoing vocation. So, we continued to support and nurture her here, and also in the opportunities that came up to explore her learning skills in a supported academic environment, which included her completion in 2018 of a diocesan foundation ministry course, her ongoing work with an Assistant Director of Ordinands, and her first year of study with the regional training course. This openness to learn has been a key element of Pat's growing ministry.

Pat has an unquenchable energy and commitment in her willingness to be a fellow traveller and in her ability to be alongside those for whom there are no answers or solutions. She is demonstrably an accompanier, alongside people at *their* pace and with their agenda, simply being there, exemplifying an outstanding model of pastoral ministry of "meeting people where they are". In the face of a complex pastoral encounter, Pat is the gentle calm, always able to be there in the changing environment of the acute human experience for which we offer a listening ear and support. A senior doctor has said he wished he could offer Pat to his patients "on prescription"! Pat has a desire to empower patients, to be with them as they grow in confidence to identify and explore whatever is needed for themselves. In short, she shows skills in both pastoral and spiritual care, identifiably in both incarnational and sacramental ministry, meaning as a gifted listener accompanier and with an ability to identify the skills and limitations in others, helping them see moments of transformation. Increasingly Pat has grown in showing her ability to teach new volunteers, encourage experienced practitioners and help the professional to recognize new insights. Further, her work, *supportive* of existing practices, has developed over time into areas of work under her own initiative, including teaching, support of pastoral visitors, and an "end-of-life" project, supporting patients, families and staff.

Developing skills in the specialist care and sensitivity of "end-of-life" pastoral visiting, Pat initially provided support on one ward as part of their "end-of-life" care project. This was based on a national project to enhance staff communication with the dying and their families and is led here by senior clinical staff. This hospital asked if we could begin to provide experienced pastoral visitors to support patients and families in this context. Pat was the first to do this here and is deeply valued in this role, continuing to nurture these skills in other experienced members of our pastoral volunteer team, while the project extends to other wards.

Pat also shared in our reflective group support of staff on the initial unit and continues in support of other pastoral visitors involved.

Pat's accompanying ministry is welcomed by everyone, including by pastoral visitor volunteers, who routinely seek her advice. She has developed the support of pastoral visitors requesting to shadow her for their own development: both new and experienced pastoral visitors have asked for, or been offered and welcomed, Pat's support to visit with them (either to shadow her work or for her to go with them to their ward) in order to work together and share skills and experiences. This has colloquially and very warmly come to be called "being Pat-tested"! This moved naturally to Pat's involvement in the development of further nurturing and teaching of pastoral visitors. To this end, we created a "Pastoral Buddy" role, meaning support provided for the novice pastoral visitor. (This is described in Chapter 4.) Whether in reflective practice, or supporting a colleague shadowing her, or else "buddying" the novice, Pat models our adventure for learning, always saying that she feels more likely to learn from her accompanying colleague than they are from her.

## One story informing others

Having the privilege to share Pat's story, as part of our *Creating Space* journey, has added to our experiences of discerning the chaplain through supporting visiting clergy and helping curates see the way ahead. In 2012–13, at the end of Jan's curacy, we developed learning outcomes for assistant ministers in hospital-based chaplaincy for the diocese. Pat's story has aided further development of this work, and in 2018 the diocese acknowledged the learning outcomes as suitable for both chaplaincy discernment and chaplaincy curacy. Before we explore further the significant issues that this has raised, in terms of the very slow progress towards seeing chaplaincy as a model of ministry beyond the parish model, we offer the learning outcomes developed here (Pearce 2018).

## Learning outcomes: grid to text

Emerging from the opportunity to support a curate moving from parish to healthcare chaplaincy was the chance to translate the "parish model" language into our context. The learning outcomes are based on those we developed for assistant ministers and *add contextually* to all that the Church's discernment process would expect otherwise. These are divided into the Church of England's nine selection criteria as set at the time of Pat's formal discernment during 2018 and course training from 2018 to 2021. However, during the 2021/22 academic year, these nine criteria, which have formed the basis of Anglican vocational discernment for nearly twenty years, will be developed instead into a model of six individual qualities assessed over four domains. This change is described as "qualities rather than criteria" that are to be "inhabited" and thus "a life-long process that is ever deepening" (Church of England 2020: 2).

The six qualities, assessed at two different stages in the diocesan stage of the applicant's discernment, firstly cover their experience and practice in areas of discipleship, mission and empowering others, and then at a later stage consider their inner life, so their personality, character and relationships. At Stage 1, the three qualities are explored over the two domains of Christ and Church, and then at Stage 2, the other three qualities are explored over the two domains of World and Self (Church of England 2020). It does rather feel as though these are focussed initially on "doing" and only much later on the candidates' "being". It will be interesting to see how this fits with the discernment of the "being" ministry of chaplaincy.

The learning outcomes developed for Pat will be duly "translated" into the new model during the time of her curacy and so the material from the older nine criteria will still provide the essence of the ongoing discernment and learning desired.

While some of the following description of the nine criteria in our context repeats work from previous chapters, this nevertheless provides in summary the way in which it was possible to add to the learning outcomes grid provided by the Ministry Division and diocese, from parish to chaplain ministry context.

## Vocation and ministry within the Church of England

Chaplaincy is a listening and accompanying ministry that "meets people where they are" (Mowat and Swinton 2007: 30), where the chaplain is a listening ear, being alongside as the other person explores solutions for themselves, and then only offers faith support if desired. This is a ministry as "chaplain standing in the world . . . and looking around" (Walters 2017: 51). It means hearing the patient's story, at their pace and their agenda. This celebrates and makes space to hear the richness of a unique human story. This is in the forum of other voices, accompanying people of every faith and none. Nevertheless, the chaplain will need to demonstrate evidence of their own tradition and faith nurture.

In addition to their sense of calling to ordained ministry, someone exploring chaplaincy will have a strong draw towards being "church" in a secular environment, where their primary focus is not a faith agenda. They will have a strong feel for this "hinterland" or "wilderness" ministry (Moody 1999: 15). In traditional language, they will be energized by working with the "unchurched", but without any agenda to bring them to faith, unless such exploration is desired by the other. They will be both aware and confident enough of their own integrity and tradition, and yet flexible enough to be challenged in faith, and to meet an eclectic and changing community of people from every faith and none, including those for whom any organized religion is a total anathema. They will have a sense of their own ongoing journeying, of the evolving nature of discerning God's call to this ministry, of the importance of learning and development. A reflective practitioner, they will demonstrate maturity, self-awareness and the ability to critically interpret experience, being both reflective and reflexive (for example Cobb 2005; Swift 2009; Bolton 2010). They will have developed a clear sense of incarnational and sacramental ministry (being alongside and identifying transformation) in the environment of acute human experience, the place of significant change and challenge.

Considering chaplaincy as a public ministry, healthcare chaplaincy is a paradigm of "public" and "practical" (*not* applied) theology. It is ministry at the interface of religion and the public space but where human need is at its most challenging. Chaplains borrow language and models from their faith background because "theology is their expertise" (Pattison 2015b: 111). It is "a source of nurture, challenge and insight" (Pattison 2015b: 126) with religion as an example and not an end in itself. Practical theology is "always contextual" (Graham et al. 2005: 10), "studying lived experience" while "holding the immediacy of praxis and narrative in creative tension" (Graham 2012: 198). All involved are changed by the pastoral encounter.

Developing learning in this area of ministry in terms of public and legal responsibilities, "occasional offices" will include emergency baptisms in challenging circumstances (for example the Emergency Department, or Neonatal ICU) and often in a pastoral context of espoused rather than normative theology and ecclesiology. Marriages will also be as an emergency, likely for a terminal patient who still has capacity, and will either be civil (chaplain-arranged with a local registrar) or requiring an archbishop's licence. Funerals will mostly be neonatal or stillbirths, while adult funerals will include the burial of those without next-of-kin. This will not include parish experience of PCCs, APCMs, Church Representation Rules or synodical government.

This ministry will include issues of governance, so confidentiality, data protection, safeguarding, DBS checks, allocation of duties/rotas and working with volunteers; it will not provide experience of church building maintenance or faculties.

In the context of public worship and preaching, additional to Eucharistic and Daily Office worship in the hospital chapel, this ministry will include bedside communion in a busy ward environment, naming and blessing of stillborn babies, occasional offices as outlined, other "civic" events such as Remembrance and memorial (adult and baby) services. It will include working and worshipping in a wide ecumenical team and alongside volunteers with no religious affinity. Congregations can include patients, staff and visitors, and can often be disrupted. It will not include school experience.

Chaplaincy ministry will mean work in a secular or polyphonic environment as generic chaplain to all faiths and none, a non-proselytizing role of ministry to patients, staff and relatives. It is a ministry of presence offering pastoral and spiritual care, often where no other role will fulfil the need. It involves roles of public conscience and advocacy, while being non-partisan. In this context, the public setting is an acutely diverse forum of the best and worst of human situations and perspectives, including views taken by those of secular, multi-faith and the host of Christian denominational perceptions. This means representing the Church in the public arena with the voice which may traditionally have offered a respected cultural and religious perspective, but now earns its place at the table by relational development, and does not assume its right to be there, but welcomes the opportunity to be a fellow guest in some contexts, as well as being the "welcoming guest" (Walton, M. 2012: 226), or else utterly rejected. It is a ministry of presence and of absence. The Emmaus Road Gospel (Luke 24:13–35) provides rich imagery for this ministry of encounter.

The majority of people served by a chaplain will be people of no faith, and there needs to be evidence in the chaplain's ministry of a willingness to explore and demonstrate the universal, yet individual, nature of spirituality and the difference between spirituality and religion. A chaplain usually works in an ecumenical team in this multi-faith environment and needs to be alert to his/her own tradition/spiritual home while being able to work alongside others of a variety of other experiences, values and beliefs.

With chaplaincy as a paradigm of practical theology, contextual storytelling alongside the development of practice (Graham et al. 2005; Graham 2012) has at its heart theological reflection. The chaplain therefore will develop key skills in reflective practice. The healthcare context, by the very nature of the patient's journey, is one that is an "insecure and uncertain landscape" requiring the ministry of one who is able "to inhabit uncertainty and change" (Swift 2009: 122, 169). Each pastoral encounter is a tool for learning because "pastoral practice not reflected upon is practice that only partially fulfils its potential" (Kelly 2010: 48). Chaplaincy research has shown that in team reflection the pastoral encounter is repeatedly the source of ongoing learning, and the reflective space itself *is* a pastoral encounter, seeing both the experiences *and* the reflective practitioners themselves as a source for learning (Pearce 2018: 150).

## Spirituality

In the developing ministry of the chaplain, it is important to be able to recognize and explore "spirituality" in this context as both universal and individual *and* as the inner place of self-awareness and searching, to make sense of oneself in one's particular situation (Mowat 2008; Swinton and Pattison 2010). Spiritual care is a significant area of ministry that involves being alongside people as they try to make sense of their situation and look for answers for themselves in their coping; it therefore involves creating space for them to do this. This will not only be demonstrated in the pastoral encounter with patients, but also within one's own team of both ordained and lay ministry, clergy and volunteers. It means giving space to listen, to speak and be heard, recognizing shared skills and personal qualities, and identifying the gifts in others. It is a collaborative environment of inviting colleagues to help "take the log out of your own eye, and then ... see clearly to take the speck out of your neighbour's eye" (Matthew 7:5).

This is a listening and accompanying ministry that "meets people where they are" (Mowat and Swinton 2007: 30), where the chaplain is a listening ear (pastoral care), being alongside as the other person explores solutions for themselves (spiritual care), and then only offers faith/religious support if desired. This is a ministry to empower others to tell their story as they try to make sense of their own situation, and to ensure that the agenda is that of the storyteller. The listener may never know the whole story, but having met in a pastoral encounter, leaves the other to go their own way and make their own discoveries. Once more, the Emmaus Road disciples offer this image of encounter, journeying, inner discovery and transformation.

A chaplain will be sufficiently confident in awareness of their own integrity and tradition to be nurtured and supported by it, and yet flexible enough to be challenged in faith. Working in an eclectic and changing community of people from every faith and none develops a holistic sense of self-development alongside the nurture and learning of others. Each will have a sense of their own ongoing journeying, of the evolving nature of discerning God's call to this ministry, a constant sense of learning and development.

The chaplain contributes to the team's "daily office" pattern and other aspects of team spiritual nurture, such as reading, study and reflection. They show evidence of personal prayer and reflection pattern.

## Personality and character

Today chaplaincy offers the public ministry that has been seen traditionally in the parish, and the open accessibility of the chaplain means they are frequently approached in the hospital by those who would never usually seek contact with clergy. It is ministry at the interface of religion and the public space, but where human need is at its most challenging. It is a ministry in the daily experience of being alongside people in crisis, equipped to work there with self-awareness, maturity, reflection and reflexivity.

Self-awareness and skills in reflective and reflexive practice are all key to the person of the chaplain. As part of a team committed to reflective practice, both personal and corporate, the curate also makes use of one-to-one reflection with their training incumbent (or mentor) and the engagement with team reflection. He/she will also engage with ongoing ministry development and all personal and professional support in healthcare and the Church. In addition, this ministry requires a distinct level of insight to be able to share personal needs and joys with colleagues.

## Relationships

Relationships will be local and corporate, secular and faith connected. In a place of acute human experience the chaplain, working generically for patients, staff and visitors in a non-proselytizing role of pastoral and spiritual care, will provide a vast arena for this experience (albeit excluding schools). It is a ministry of presence.

In an environment of acute human experience (change and challenge), the chaplain will have regular experience of meeting people who are in a place of crisis and will only be ably equipped to work alongside such situations if they possess self-awareness, maturity and reflexivity.

In addition to recognizing the value of good practice in pastoral and professional relationships, the chaplain will also be able to work alongside others of a variety of other experiences and beliefs, and working in the environment of acute human experience will supply a great deal of material for this.

## Leadership and collaboration

This ministry will, most effectively, involve the care of a number of volunteers but in a rather more diverse area of work than the parish church. The chaplain will be able to work creatively in and contribute to a mixed team of both clergy and laity, including volunteers in both, where reflective practice should be both personal and corporate. The chaplain will be able to assimilate and share their own existing professional skills. They will also be able to share in the nurture of a large number of volunteers in a variety of roles, including supporting them to develop their own and others' skills as a reflective practitioner.

Healthcare chaplaincy ministry includes experience in other forms of multi-disciplinary teams including clinical and non-clinical, practitioners and trainees. This is another aspect of the public ministry role where, for the chaplain-reflective-practitioner, "theology is their expertise", as "a source of nurture, challenge and insight" (Pattison 2015b: 111, 126) with religion as an example and not an end in itself. This background, personally and professionally, is a developing resource, equipping the chaplain to work with self-awareness, maturity, reflection and reflexivity alongside others, empowering *their* use and development of these skills in context.

The chaplain will also have the ability to be both self-motivated and yet able to discern need for advice or support. They will be able to reflect on their understanding of work in a healthcare environment and consider comparisons with parish ministry, as well as being able to recognize accountability to both Church and healthcare authorities. They will be able to empower others and contribute to the team in the constructive support of all.

## Mission and evangelism

If mission is "what we do" and evangelism is "how we go about it", then healthcare chaplaincy's mission, in context, is to "live the Gospel" by being alongside people, journeying with them as they make their own discoveries through reflection and insight, like on the Emmaus Road (Luke 24:13-35). This is demonstrated in pastoral and spiritual care, with faith care if desired. An alternative image is the manifestation of the Great Commandment (Matthew 22:36-40, rehearsed in Common Worship Holy Communion), to love God and neighbour. While recognizing the Church of England's Five Marks of Mission (tell, teach, tend, transform, treasure), the emphasis nevertheless of "being" rather than "doing" is important here. The ability to see the difference between parish and chaplaincy ministry includes different emphasis on faith provision and nurture. Where faith support *has* been desired or appropriate, clearly this is at the request, the agenda, pace and route, of the other person in the encounter. The chaplaincy role is not to proselytize (NHS Chaplaincy Guidelines 2015: 9).

In the team, in the chaplain's own self-care, and where appropriate elsewhere, theological reflection may explore identifying God's presence in the broken places of human experiences. This, as has been described, is then the root competence for developing insight and skill in the pastoral encounter. In turn, developing skills in the pastoral encounter nurtures the pastoral and spiritual care of the other person present, whether patient, staff or otherwise.

Being part of the Church in a multi-phonic environment, chaplaincy ministry is to accompany, "meeting people where they are", with pastoral care as the listening to their story and spiritual care as supporting the patient while they find answers themselves in their situation. The chaplain, working generically for patients, staff and visitors in a non-proselytizing role of pastoral and spiritual care, recognizes that provision for religious need will be mostly reactive. Proactive faith nurture and support will be either subsequent to this, or as part of identifiable public and corporate work of the worshipping life of the chaplaincy department, and in the nurture of colleagues and volunteers. This is discipleship by "being", meaning *responding to* rather than actively seeking out.

This ministry explores human experience at this moment and in this context. Active connection with "contemporary culture", whether in relation to faith or not, and in whatever context, is essential in this ministry as "chaplain in the world ... and looking around" (Walters 2017: 51). It is a ministry of presence, responding to people's situations. "Meeting people where they are" also means responding to those who seek faith support, in their context, agenda, pace and route. This will be at the request of the other person in the pastoral encounter, and will require acute sensitivity to the reality of the challenge of the patient's context and to any existing, or desired, relationship with the local church. Contribution to faith development will also be true for the life and nurture of the eclectic chaplaincy team.

The healthcare environment is pluralistic and provides encounter with people of all ages and from every life circumstance. Where preaching and formal teaching is appropriate, whether involving patients, staff, volunteers and visitors, it will be sensitive to the impact on them of the environment of challenge and change.

## Faith and quality of mind

In healthcare, a willingness to engage with people of every faith and none is essential, as well as a whole variety of Christian traditions. Any preaching and teaching will be sensitive to the context. Additional to specific expectations of exegetical knowledge and hermeneutical insights in the context of today's world and daily living, the chaplain should nurture this in the context of acute human need, as their own supportive resource. This reveals the evolving nature of discerning God's call to ministry, being reflective and reflexive, in the face of acute human experience. Depending on the culture of the chaplaincy team, this may include weekday and Sunday preaching, contributions to volunteer reflection, and seasonally led reflective study sessions such as Advent and Lent. This work will not provide the breadth of scriptural engagement possible in the parish worshipping community, but the pastoral connections will be significant.

As has been described, the chaplain's professional and personal development will require being committed to reflective practice, both personal and corporate, and engaging with all means of support for personal and professional development both in healthcare and the Church. Working creatively in a mixed team of both clergy and laity, including volunteers in both, they will be alert to the nurture of both themselves and others. Alert to occasions of applied theology but mostly public and practical theology, the chaplain works.

In their ministry the chaplain will encounter almost every life circumstance and acute human experience. Each pastoral encounter will be significant, occurring, for example, in the face of life-changing challenge, loss of control, a change in life choices or being faced with death, including that of a baby.

Here, reflecting together will combine developments in areas of both faith and quality of mind. Working and reflecting within the ecumenical team in a multi-faith environment, alert to one's own tradition/spiritual home but able to work alongside others of a variety of other experiences, values and beliefs, and working in the environment of acute human experience, will supply a great deal of material for this.

## Summary reflections on "learning outcomes"

Thus far we have explored the ways in which sharing our experiences as chaplains with others, including parish clergy and curates as well as pastoral visitor volunteers, has informed both them and us. We have explored our experiences of discerning the chaplain both within and beyond the hospital. We have shown how, by adding to the existing parish model, we can identify specific chaplaincy skills that help identify someone with a vocation to this unique ministry. We share now further reflections offering a way ahead for the wider Church.

## Chaplain vocational discernment

More recently, there has been a glimmer of willingness for the Church to recognize that there are different shapes of ministries that could be discerned early on in the ordinand's training process. However, that is insufficient unless early discernment seeks to incorporate this notion as a new norm. For some time, there have been suggestions that simply imagining that potential ordinands, or any clergy for that matter, should be fitted into a prescribed parish-shaped model, is inadequate and inappropriate. Instead, we should be looking down the other end of the telescope at applicants' gifts, skills and potential to determine what type of ministry could benefit from these, as Thornton (2013) discusses in a lecture entitled "Character and Charism". Of course, once discernment to chaplaincy *as primary ministry* becomes more prevalent, it will be regarded as less of a deviation from the norm and with rather more familiarity. Already there are chaplains who have completed their curacy in this way (models include part parish/part chaplaincy or concluding curacy in a chaplaincy after a period in a parish). We have been aware of at least one final year student and an ordinand whose curacy was expected to be exclusively grounded in chaplaincy, and to be documented as such; yet for our curate parish hours have been made mandatory.

## Ordination training

When Jan was ordained for ministry ten years ago, there was no mention of initial vocation to chaplaincy. There was an explicit assumption that we were all going to work in parishes. Perhaps there was a passing nod that we might be called to a different shape of ministry in the future, but that was definitely not something to consider at the start of one's ordained life. Because curacy had always been seen as parish-based from discernment onwards, training was unlikely to reflect any departure from that norm. Of course, almost all ordination training is relevant to whatever setting we find ourselves in, but on reflection, there was a yawning gap, an opportunity to recognize ministry in different forms. Surely this would help parish-based ordinands and clergy in general to understand and value the role of chaplains and therefore to honour and recognize that particular ministry?

If there is recognition that ordinands are going to be able to serve their curacies in a chaplaincy (or elsewhere), then it is not only discernment that needs to encompass this, but likewise ordination training. It is not enough to speak in training about "when you get to your parishes" and then casually mention alternatives like chaplaincy as an afterthought. What is taught in ordination training is highly relevant for chaplaincy but is almost always taught from the angle of a parish-based context, when it need not be. Increasingly, ordinands will be studying alongside those who will and those who will not be serving in a parish, and it is important that the "parish default model" attitude is relinquished.

If the historical assumption that "parish" is the only way forward becomes redundant, then we can start envisioning chaplaincy ministry (and other forms) as of equal worth and importance. The myth that chaplaincy is the "poor relation" of parish ministry has to go; this envisioning needs to be encouraged and embraced by clergy at all levels of seniority. The language that has historically been used to describe non-parish ministry is at best discouraging: the words "secular", "sector" and "marginal", even if accurate, hardly invoke a sense of equality, value and positive recognition.

The overriding perception that chaplaincy ministry is something that comes only after a parish curacy is also echoed today:

> Some people serve in Chaplaincy settings—for example hospitals, schools, prisons, armed forces and whilst a curacy might enable you to explore this to some extent, it is after curacy you can really consider doing this as the sole focus of ministry (from <https://www.peterborough-diocese.org.uk/>, accessed 6 May 2021).

Nevertheless, there are moves to allow curacies to take place in chaplaincies. The *Church Times* General Synod report (1 March 2019) in referring to Amending Canon 39 reported "another change would allow ordinands to be ordained not as an assistant curate in a particular parish but to a Bishop's Mission initiative or a non-parochial institution". However, despite all efforts and initial understandings, our own curate was obliged to prepare for her curacy to be combined, meaning based in healthcare chaplaincy but also having some regular element of parish experience.

Having so far outlined our further case for healthcare chaplaincy as a distinct and discernible ministry to which many may be called without any parish work, we develop our *Creating Space* story by identifying ministry in the hospital and outside during a time of national and international crisis in terms of the COVID-19 pandemic.

CHAPTER 9

# Living with a virus

While the COVID-19 pandemic has infected not only people's health but our whole way of life, so it has turned up discoveries in the most unexpected and unlikely places. The familiar words "kindness of strangers" may describe something of these discoveries. In Tennessee Williams' play the tragic Blanche DuBois declares, as her life takes another distressing turn, the value of "the kindness of strangers" (Williams 1957: 107), the help along the way from people she does not know. The phrase appears in a number of places, for example in the titles of films, a television series, a journalist's autobiography (Adie 2002) and a book of travel stories of connecting with others, the support in and from the unfamiliar (O'Nuallain 2018). It has come to mean the unexpected comfort from unlikely places. The pandemic context has and remains such a journey of discovery, just as " ... the wanderer depends on the kindness of strangers" (Child 1997: 57). In the first of Lee Child's "Jack Reacher" stories, Jack disembarks from the cross-country bus, apparently on a whim, in the middle of nowhere. Yet, in happening to be there, he discovers that this is where his estranged brother has just died. He also finds that he becomes the friend of several local people who are in need of his skills, as well as discovering himself being nurtured by the care of those he has never met before. Indeed, the story is about a new and transient community of strangers who, for a period of time, bring vital help and support to each other before they part company, step out on the road ahead and go their own way.

Our "Creating Space" story has many similar elements, in the meeting of strangers, the chance encounter in the landscape of change and uncertainty, being alongside those who are suddenly facing crisis and ongoing challenge. In the spring of 2020, this was of course true of the COVID-19 pandemic for all healthcare staff, patients and families. As healthcare chaplains, we are clearly not alone in our experiences, recognizing that colleagues elsewhere in the country, and across the world, will have had a more complex and demanding time than we may have experienced. However, we share here as chaplains and practical theologians our story and reflections on our experiences in our context, in the belief that reading the reflections of strangers can encourage others to look further at their own story.

In this chapter, we offer various vignettes of our pastoral encounters, narratives drawn together to demonstrate supporting staff through these pandemic months. We outline one of the early experiences at the start of the lockdown in deciding to stop providing bedside communion temporarily: how we reached this decision, what this felt like, and how we would present this to a patient seeking this sort of faith care. We highlight experiences of the unseen benefits of having to do things differently. We describe the ways in which much of our day-to-day ministry changed in terms of needing to provide remote support to families unable to visit, including those facing bereavement, as well as staff working in new places, often feeling that they were facing another whole new stratosphere of change and challenge, feeling constantly on the back foot. On occasion we felt our work was merely vaguely, remotely, supporting! In this chapter, we also offer reflections from colleagues of their own experiences including during weeks when we had asked our volunteers to stand down and we, as a team of four salaried chaplains, were working on a 50/50 basis with two on site and two working from home. We draw out experiences of doing things differently, meaning exploring, even daily from the very start of the virus outbreak, how our department and routine practices would evolve. The COVID-19 pandemic is a significant example of the practical theology of the experiences of the familiar, that is, seeing daily the taken-for-granted practice that is then explored, to "know the place for the first time" (Eliot 1944: 43), and the praxis that evolves into the new normal. This exemplifies being constantly mindful that the contextual dialogue of narrative and praxis (Graham 2005, 2012) can be a moment-by-moment journey on a road, "the one less travelled by" (Frost 2017: 7).

## Pastoral encounters: supporting staff in a pandemic year

Continuing to find ways to offer support to staff throughout this pandemic, we have regularly reported our empirical data of staff pastoral encounters to the hospital's staff wellbeing steering group. The figures include any member of staff being in meaningful conversation with a member of our team and this happening in a whole variety of contexts. Our data has shown that we have seen from forty to sixty staff per month during the year March 2020 to March 2021.

Regardless of time or context, in these encounters we "create space", meaning to listen to whatever it may be that the person finds they would like to talk about. By listening, we are alongside staff while they think about how they are dealing with whatever may be their experiences or thoughts at the time. Some find that a one-off chat in confidence, one-to-one with any of us, is just the space they need. For others, it may be over several visits, or for as long as they like. This is entirely their choice, whatever they feel is most helpful. Equally, a staff encounter can also be a conversation in the corridor or on their ward/unit. We are available for staff support, one-to-one or in a group, face-to-face or on the telephone, twenty-four hours a day. While this has always been true, in one way or another for the life of this department, actually articulating the offer of telephone support for distressed staff overnight has only really been actively highlighted amid the pandemic year. During this time, a number of staff warmly expressed surprise and comfort from knowing there was a listening ear available twenty-four hours a day.

While still informal, the more structured support we offer staff is in group reflections called "Space for Wellbeing". Not only in the pandemic context, and alongside our one-to-one space for staff, this is part of our ongoing practice, mirroring the staff support highlighted in Chapter 3, evolving from Sacha's research. As outlined then, this became, and continues to be, a key element in our support of staff teams and groups. "Space for Wellbeing" is space for reflection, using our own simple, short reflective cycle, with a small group of staff, from their ward or unit or other team base. This lasts about thirty minutes and can happen either on their ward/unit/usual work environment, or in our department. It is space to talk about, explore and learn from their experiences, discovering how to be both professional and human, as a whole person, in their team relationships and in their own particular context. This kind of staff support is well known across our staff and management so, as the virus took hold during 2020, a variety of healthcare leaders asked us to offer "our reflective support" to staff at the coalface of "red wards" and intensive care units where the acute COVID-19 patients were being treated. This was available daily for "red wards", advertised for two half-hour sessions morning and afternoon based on the timing of the staff work pattern and their hours in full PPE. In this case, the staff were invited daily by their manager, if they chose, to attend these sessions, which were deliberately held off the ward so they were able to get away from their work environment. This was an interesting opportunity to explore because, both within Sacha's research and in our usual practice, these reflective sessions are more usually held within the ward/unit space in order to make the sessions accessible, easy to arrange and for staff to return to work if needed urgently. A similar offer of regular reflective space was provided on particular days and times in the week for critical care staff within their units. Both during the acute phases of the pandemic, and as numbers began to reduce, we were also invited to wards/teams where change had meant physically moving all staff and patients to another ward/unit. We met the face of acute change and challenge alongside both the clinical and support staff, in doorways, in corridors, in meeting rooms, outside PPE changing rooms, or within the "red zone" itself.

## Vignettes of pastoral encounters with staff as we live together with a virus

To some extent, the COVID-19 experience has raised a number of the familiar staff issues, such as a particular work-related stressful issue or experience, which then opens up into talking about deeper personal concerns. However, the pandemic has brought another kind of challenge, most usually related to issues such as uncertainty, change, fear and exhaustion. From each pastoral encounter with staff, whether one-to-one or in a group, the frequent response is of gratitude for our time and twenty-four-hour availability, and for space to be heard without judgement.

The most vivid of reflections from staff have included those deeply affected by the number of deaths they witnessed in a relatively short period of time. There have been a few descriptions from staff looking back over the pandemic months, feeling tearful, remembering patients who were scared, gasping for breath, reaching out and gasping as they died. In several scenarios there has been the sense of "being on the front line", where the conflict analogy was not difficult to see. Overall, through support and reflection, this has clearly been a mammoth learning experience for everyone, personally and professionally.

The staff quotations in the rest of this section were gathered from a wide selection from those contributing anonymously to the hospital reflections after the 2020/2021 first year.

> In the first lockdown I couldn't go to work, and felt isolated, and it was as though I wasn't helping, wasn't making a difference. I guess I was feeling guilty for shielding. I'm really glad I can make my contribution now though.

For some, the issues relate to coming back into the hospital environment after a period of perhaps being unwell themselves or for having had reasons to isolate. On returning to work, there has been a sense of feeling traumatized and completely unable to engage with colleagues or patients. We have supported staff who, feeling the need to go home, feeling physically unable to be in the hospital building, were directed by their manager to us, and after talking felt able to return to their workplace.

Other staff described feeling upset and anxious on their first day back after a period of working remotely. Drawing together several scenarios, while staff spoke of the hospital as a safe place to work, some recounted that working from home brought its own sense of isolation. In some contexts, staff felt unprepared, untrained and alone with immense responsibility, saying that if they were working in the hospital, they could have found advice on how best to proceed. At home, perhaps dealing with a difficult telephone call, say with a patient or relative, the experience felt more personal and precarious. For some, working at home can mean carrying the stress alone but also a sense of foreboding in returning to the hospital. In a few narratives, there was a feeling that the whole COVID-19 experience had become inevitably such a priority that other, more personal needs were worsened by fearing they would be ignored. On several occasions, staff came to us at the point of going home and found space and time to reflect on the impact of their experiences and to better understand them. Such opportunities as these regularly end with staff feeling an overwhelming pressure or stress being lifted or released and being able afterwards to return to work rather than go home.

There have been groups of staff who have asked for support who have felt very unsettled because of the change in their working context and the relocation of some of their team. As the COVID-19 numbers began to reduce in 2021, there was a feeling among many of being glad to be back, or going back, to their familiar ward/unit to work. Equally, others felt exhausted and nervous of starting back in the "normal" environment, feeling there had not been enough time to process their experiences. In all these scenarios, reflecting with a chaplain gave them space to talk together and work through some challenging professional and personal issues. Their thanks were expressed in their unanimous gratitude for having space to talk.

A member of staff came to see our department asking to reflect on several personal issues, but also with concerns in their working environment. Already learning to live with several areas of personal anxiety, they expressed concerns in working in "red zones", meaning wards with patients with a COVID-19 diagnosis. Their feelings were that there were not enough staff to deal with the workload as well as to help with PPE. After one session with a chaplain, and although they described being well supported by their immediate manager, they felt that they would like to return in a couple of weeks in order to have somewhere to talk over their anxiety and concerns.

On another occasion someone came to the department in a state of deep distress. They do not usually work where they were that day but had volunteered to work there during the first lockdown period. A member of their own family had been admitted elsewhere with COVID-19 and subsequently died. They found this traumatic event very difficult to manage. Grateful for somewhere to go to talk about their distress, their subsequent occasional "meltdowns" at work mean they have seen a chaplain for support at these times.

> I would like to thank everyone for how they treated my relative. But I want them to remember that they were not a statistic, a number; their life mattered and their passing has left a huge gap in our lives.

Within a matter of days of each other, three healthcare professional specialist teams, each independent of the other, approached us looking for "Space for Wellbeing" reflective support for their group. The manager of one group, who felt overwhelmed by the amount of "listening ear" they were providing in their office, came looking for help for themselves and their team. They described staff coming to them in tears, feeling swamped, exhausted with their work. For another team, this was a repeat request, having used our reflective method before, inviting us to return to their team as they had begun to feel individually isolated in their work pattern, with no opportunity to connect and support each other. For the third group, the request was related to a sense of being overwhelmed emotionally as a result of their COVID-19 related work and looking for somewhere, and some way, to find support and an opportunity to learn.

A member of staff came to our department one day looking for somewhere to talk. For several reasons they had had to be redeployed from their usual place of work and been given other employment elsewhere within the Trust. They expressed a strong desire to return to their previous role and a desperate need to access support during that period of time, which they felt was made more difficult to find while there was a greater focus on COVID-19 issues. During their one-to-one with a chaplain, this person was able to explore what they were able to achieve in their present situation and what they hope for in the future, as well as reflect on their own feelings at that time. This was the space they had been seeking.

A member of staff contacted the duty chaplain by telephone one weekend. They were upset and fearful of coming to work the next day. They and their family had recently had the COVID-19 virus and were still coping with the after-effects of the illness. Although the caller had already returned to work from sick leave, they were not looking forward to a new working week, feeling upset and conflicted on a number of levels. They did not want to take more time off work. They wanted to try and "stay in it" in order to care for critically ill COVID-19 patients in their care. They wanted to continue to be a support to their colleagues, who were already under great pressure with others still off work. Although they wanted to work, each time they were on shift, they recognized they felt vulnerable. They were tearful, emotional, worried for the patients and afraid for themselves, and felt under pressure "to get over it and get on with it". At the end of the telephone call, a one-to-one session was arranged for Monday morning face-to-face with the same chaplain. The telephone conversation and the one-to-one the next day provided a first real opportunity to have the time and safe space to reflect upon recent events and discern the best way forward. The offer of future sessions was gratefully appreciated. The member of staff decided they would not take any further time off, would continue to work, very aware that if things got difficult, they knew they had somewhere to go to talk further.

One chaplain describes visiting a ward/unit and encountering several members of staff who, while busy, were keen to pause for a moment to talk. They expressed a mix of emotions, many looking tired and some even near to tears. Some felt they were "doing their bit" although facing a higher level of professional challenge. Others described a sort of resilience, the need to "keep calm and carry on", that if they thought about their work for too long, they would be unable to keep going. Throughout, there was a strong feeling of gratitude that they had been given a few moments to talk.

Gathering examples from several "Space for Wellbeing" reflective sessions, staff from different "red zone" contexts, and at different times, described a whole variety of feelings across both negative and positive themes. For many there was greater uncertainty about what each shift in the "red zone" and in PPE would bring, and for some there was a fear of being alone and unsupported, even feeling stretched and unable to deliver a high enough standard of care. Some spoke of feeling forced to make very challenging choices or concerned that other staff would be prioritizing which patient would get the best level of care. Some felt that under pressure they were doing things for which they had little or no experience, or else that they were struggling under unrelenting pressure and exhaustion in a constant work cycle. One healthcare professional said, "It's like you've run a marathon!" Some described feeling unable to get a drink when you needed one, or use the bathroom, of constantly feeling hot, dehydrated and trapped. At the beginning of each cycle of hours behind closed doors in the "red zone", a few said they were afraid of what they would find "when you go back in". However, there were those who described feeling proud to work professionally on the front line of the COVID-19 pandemic. There were those who welcomed the opportunity for new experiences and professional development. Several spoke of enjoying working in new teams where the work was particularly focussed, with the emphasis on getting it done and being in it together. In this context also, some said that not knowing each other very well actually helped them focus on the work.

> I'm constantly exhausted, emotionally and physically. But others seem to revel in the challenges. There is no such thing as "normal" anymore.

> I only qualified during the first lockdown. It's been horrendous. I worked on a red ward and in one shift seven people died there. But the support from colleagues has kept me, kept us all going.

> It's hard to sum up the past year really. It's too much pain everywhere, separation from loved ones, constant change at work, the risk of taking the virus home. But there is hope for the future, whatever that is.

As chaplains and healthcare staff, we share this landscape of change and uncertainty, being alongside one another as those who are suddenly facing crisis and ongoing challenge. However, as we reflect, it is clear that there is so much to be learnt, endeavouring to make sense of letting go of the familiar and finding new grounds for discovery in our human experience.

## Using practical theology: bedside communion to spiritual communion

As we have explored, healthcare chaplaincy is a rich paradigm of practical theology in the changing and challenging hinterland of acute human experience. Early in the *Creating Space* story, a powerful image of practical theology, on which we reflected for a number of years, was the request on several occasions to baptize a dying baby, whose parents said they did not have any particular faith but would like this chance for their child. The thread throughout was our own existing theology, the doctrine or tradition from which we come, as we arrive in this new place, meaning the context in which we now, today, at this moment, find ourselves. Most of us as chaplains would probably baptize this child regardless, perhaps describing our action as responding to a pastoral need or demonstrating God's welcome and inclusive love for all. This may possibly be contrary to our previous parish church policy, or else the experience invites us to look again at our wider view of baptism and see what this profoundly moving experience has given us.

Practical theology is developed in dialogue with *what we already know* and *where we are now*. It is always created with the thread of existing practice (what we already know and do) but in the light of the current story, today's experience, we allow our understanding to evolve potentially into developing new practice. The liberal theologian would claim it is following in the footsteps of the divine!

Bedside communion, in the face of COVID-19, is today's vivid example. Some chaplaincy departments withdrew early on, while we were, for a while, still willing to continue providing it. Some London hospital chaplains had described placing the host (the bread) on a paper towel and offering it to the COVID-19 patient via the patient's table, so that they could pick it up themselves. However, there has also been some debate about anointing, and that this should not happen, as it means being too close to the patient and indeed near their face. On reflection, we decided to stop providing bedside communion in the current situation. These reflections, using practical theology, will show how we reached that point.

Our context is today's COVID-19 pandemic, with everyone asked to social distance. More specifically, it is in the more intense environment of the hospital, working closely with patients and staff, where COVID-19 is both an invisible and a very visible risk. This is our context, and our "lived experience" is being asked both by patients and parish clergy to offer the sacrament. The story, the narrative, takes us further, asking how we can combine these two issues: the desire to fulfil the faith expectation alongside the healthcare risk. Do we need to develop our practice? However careful we may be, in terms of taking a host (the bread) out of the pyx and placing it in an envelope or paper towel, there is no guarantee of not spreading the virus, however carefully we have washed hands or proceed with ward-based infection control protocol. In healthier times, post-virus, it may be that we do develop a practice of single use (one host/bread, one envelope) means of taking bedside communion to one patient at a time. However, what are we to do now? How do we hold "the immediacy of praxis and narrative in creative tension" (Graham 2012: 198)? In the light of the current story, we need to change our practice, meaning allowing the story to evolve our praxis.

Our decision was to withhold bedside communion until further notice, even to patients on non-COVID-19 wards, but to use the prayers of spiritual communion, a very beautiful way of inviting both the chaplain and recipient into the same place of communion with God, although this can also be done by someone alone. Specific prayers have been produced from a variety of sources inviting the praying person to be refreshed in their sense of God within them.

We have looked at our context, and at our particular experience, and held together both the story we are hearing, what's right in front of us, and our usual practice. Practical theology has helped us understand how and why we need to evolve and develop new practice, but without losing sight of the divine imperative!

The same paradigm, our modelling of practical theology, has had a similar effect on subsequent occasions through this year, other instances where the pandemic has forced us to do things differently and once again where the benefit has surprised us. Among all the church closures, and the use of broadcasting, recording or streaming worship, the social distancing of public liturgy had become all too familiar through 2020.

As guidelines eased towards the end of the year, the means of offering Holy Communion safely had been adopted by many Christian traditions. However, the announcement of the first lockdown came in the middle of Lent 2020, meaning that Ash Wednesday 2021 presented a new question of how to provide the Imposition of Ashes without touching anyone. Various traditions offered their guidelines, such as tipping ash on to the recipient at the end of the service as they left the building. This felt inappropriate in the hospital, but applying the same reflective process as we had when we adopted "spiritual communion", we discovered a method that had significant theological and, quite frankly, emotional impact. After some thought, we decided that individual portions of ashes placed on paper towels would be placed on a table at the front of the chapel, and after suitable prayers, those present would come forward at a two-metre distance from one another, collect their ashes and return to their seats. At the celebrant's words, "Remember that you are dust" they then simultaneously imposed the ash with a cross on their own foreheads. Although a very simple move, the impact of adding ash to your own forehead, being reminded that you indeed will return to dust, uncovered a palpable sense of human and personal mortality but of God's presence there. This overwhelming feeling brought a sense of taking responsibility myself for "turning away from sin and being faithful to Christ".

Our reflections move now from these examples of practical theology, as the way to help evolve our practice, to other ways in which we have explored, embraced and developed in this particular changing context.

## Remote support: being remotely supportive to wayfarers

During each of the COVID-19 lockdowns, some of the wayfarers we already support were keen to continue to receive contact from our chaplaincy team. Although they might have preferred face-to-face contact, this has not been possible due to restrictions on attending the hospital, or their own vulnerability.

The wayfarer "Jean", mentioned in Chapter 4, reported that she felt very supported with weekly, prearranged telephone calls lasting about forty-five minutes. The underlying point of these calls was, as usual, from the pastoral point of view, an opportunity to offer space for Jean to talk about the things that had been challenging for her that week. She also mentioned that the sense of support these regular contacts gave her meant she knew I would be calling; it was something for her to look forward to, and she found it helpful to share with me about how she had managed a particular challenge that week. For example, on week one, she explained that simply opening her front door was frightening, because the pandemic had contributed to her already existing fear of going out. However, on week two, knowing she would be getting a telephone call from us, she worked hard at not only opening her front door for a few minutes but actually walking down the road to pick up a parcel. It was important to her to know someone would be there on the end of the telephone to hear of her success. She felt strengthened and enabled to increase this kind of activity, because someone was interested enough to hear about it and help her consolidate her progress. As we approach the first anniversary of lockdown one, our phone calls are fortnightly, and Jean has progressed to regular socially distanced walks with a neighbour. She reports how much she values the contact with us during these restrictions on meeting and chatting with people, but the walks have also built her confidence and developed her enjoyment of a new daily activity.

Another wayfarer who was contacted solely by email (because telephoning was more problematic) replied and reported that it was very helpful to realize she had not been forgotten and that someone was there for her to contact, if only by email. Because through email we "left the door open", she then subsequently felt able to request telephone support. Others also regularly email or telephone us with their news and updates, probably much more than usual because of the isolation surrounding COVID.

A third wayfarer was also gratified to receive telephone contact, but also enjoyed sending us electronic photographs she had taken whilst on her walks. In isolation, here was someone to talk with, and while conversation was primarily about the photographs, this led to opportunities for further exploration of the wayfarer's own wellbeing during the challenges of the virus lockdown. Again, the means of pastoral support, dictated partly by the virus and each wayfarer's own particular circumstances, meant that they all reported feeling that "someone was there" for them.

This provided us with useful evidence about how pastoral support can work even in the absence of face-to-face meetings and lack of non-verbal cues. Despite our forced departure from usual practice, we were able to see how telephone support worked in action and, whilst not perhaps the optimum way of being pastoral, it was a much better option than no contact at all. But rather than simply being seen as being second best, it no doubt provided us with additional learning about being pastoral when all the obvious cues and conditions of meeting in person were not available or possible. Once again, the pandemic teaches us new things we may have never discovered.

## Remote support for patients, staff and relatives

Early in the lockdown we were approached by our bereavement department, who had begun to support families remotely by telephone and also by electronic transfer of death certificates. Their early reflections included recognizing how much families appreciated not having to come back into the hospital to collect paperwork, and that this practice may well continue post COVID-19 era. As the bereavement team worked on the telephone to families, who had been unable to visit their terminally ill relatives, it became noticeable that a space had opened in terms of communication with the hospital and that people wanted to talk. We were invited, in such cases and with the consent of the families, to call them ourselves and pick up their story. As chaplains, in our own way and in differing situations, we had each had pastoral encounter conversations on the telephone before. However, this was a different opportunity to explore a remote bereavement encounter in a new context. Our reflections included considering how to allow silence without being aware of the other person's responses, such as facial expression or body language. In every case, relatives were grateful to have someone to talk through their experiences with. For some, a single chat was enough, and for others, we were invited to ring back several times. In a strange way, this sort of bereavement support felt both new and yet familiar. We *do* include in our funeral ministry the need sometimes to have bereavement conversations and funeral planning on the telephone, or to support a family in the hospital while having nothing to do with officiating at the funeral. Yet during this time we were both remote, meaning distanced by being on the telephone, and also staying as strangers with no physical presence involvement at any time.

## "How COVID-19 changed the hospital"

Our chaplain colleague, Simon, reports on his experience and reflections:

The COVID-19 virus changed the whole environment in which a pre-pandemic society operates. In the face of scientific data projecting hundreds of thousands of deaths if nothing was done, and a health service overwhelmed with patients, the Health Service prepared as best they could for the unknown. Clinical staff were re-assigned. Wards were cleared and set up to receive COVID-19 patients. Our hospital in the south-west of England had only forty per cent occupancy at one point in March 2020, when it routinely has ninety to 104 per cent bed occupancy, and when it is only designed to run at eighty per cent.

The visiting regime was changed so that no visitors were on site at all except in the case of patients in their last days of life, one birthing partner for maternity or one parent per sick child. There has been some relaxation in the case of "end-of-life", allowing more than one visitor. Husbands, wives and close relatives all had to suffer separation, and patients felt cut off. Relatives felt disempowered and impotent, unable to help or be near loved ones. People were told of death by phone call and offered pastoral support over the phone from a team set up to offer these services.

The effect on chaplaincy visiting has been profound. Very early, before the lockdown, it was recognized that we could no longer allow volunteer visitors to go onto wards. The age profile of our pastoral volunteers was mostly over sixty and therefore potentially high risk. There was also the potential for passing on the infection from one patient to another as they moved between bed spaces. Public worship services were suspended, and on a nationwide chaplaincy email discussion group there was much conversation about whether or not to distribute Holy Communion to hospital patients. Very early, before Church authorities forbade it, we had decided not to take Communion to the bedside, since the risk of carrying infection to or from a patient was deemed to be too high. For many churchgoing patients and staff, this was completely unprecedented. Catholics had a Sunday Obligation to attend Mass, so many felt a deep sense of loss at this suspension. However, the morning Eucharist continued, not as a publicly attended service but so that it could be broadcast over hospital radio, as it always has been in our hospital.

Hospital patients who would normally have access to registrars for emergency marriages were unable to do this because of the pandemic. To address this pastoral need, a service of Love and Commitment was conducted at home for a young adult who was at the end of life. A wedding dress, already purchased for the planned marriage, was used and rings were exchanged. Of course, it did not have the force of law to be a legal marriage, but it was important for the couple at that time to express their love in front of family.

At the time of death, social isolation meant that those who were bereaved could not have non-cohabiting family members or friends visit to offer support or solace. Phone calls and video contact were better than nothing, but this was not human contact, not a hug, nor a face-to-face smile. Lack of contact was also a factor for those members of staff who were self-isolating for reasons of their own or their loved ones' health. In a Human Resources exercise to reach out to contact the two hundred-plus members of staff in this particular circumstance, isolation was very much a frequent topic of conversation, as was boredom and a feeling that staff at home were letting down their colleagues left at work. Uncertainty for the future was also evident as a cause of concern. "How will it ever be safe for me to return to work again?" was a very common question.

One particular issue was the question of whether chaplains should enter red zones where COVID-19 patients were being treated. Would it be a vital support to staff and patients, or a hindrance? Would it be a misuse of limited PPE (personal protective equipment) and would remote chaplaincy be a better option to support those inside the red zones? There were mixed opinions on these and other topics.

Going into a red zone for the first time was surreal: entering a place where there are potentially invisible infectious grenades which are anxious to infect you is a novel experience for one who has worked in and freely moved around the hospital over a number of years. Seeing and being with staff, who freely assent to working there, is also humbling. How is it they feel no fear? Do they not watch the news and see how many hospital staff are dying? The reality is that many are anxious, and the effects of these working environments on people's wellbeing and mental health may be with us for years. As I put on the surgical gown, gloves, mask, eye protection, I wondered if it made me feel safe or just reminded me how vulnerable I was. It was surprising that there were staff present without PPE, sitting behind desks, chatting, calling relatives, laughing, being "normal". Only staff approaching patients wore PPE. At the height of our infections, one red zone received more than three hundred calls per day from relatives anxious for news. A liaison person was placed on the wards. Their job was to call a nominated relative with updates: "patient sat up", "had a drink", "walked for the first time today", "sadly not responding to treatment", and pass on whatever was appropriate. Relatives craved news, and by passing this on regularly, incoming calls were reduced to thirty per day.

Speaking to a sick person through mask and visor was hard. It was hot as well. From the patients' perspective, they never see anyone's face. It must be like living in a film set, with everyone dressed up, never seeing a smile, never recognizing faces—that's "normal" and what we do as humans, but not in these circumstances.

Taking off the kit in the proper order was just as essential as putting it on correctly, including washing and using hand sanitizer. The process has been well reported and shown on TV, but it is a very personal moment. Perhaps familiarity would remove these fears—but never forget that sometimes things are very safe until you forget they are dangerous.

Naturally as the pandemic year of 2020 moved on and then changed into 2021 and a third lockdown, we all got used to living with the COVID-19 situation. Living with it meant that going onto red wards was no longer a new experience and became "routine", something that became "normal". The hospital was trying to allow relatives to be with their COVID-19 loved ones when it became clear that they were dying.

Many such "end-of-life" patients had loved ones by their bedside. For those that could not visit, possibly because they were clinically vulnerable or had the virus themselves, there was an increasing use of virtual contact. Electronic devices were used to connect patients and relatives. One of the roles of the chaplain in those situations was to be at the bedside with such a device and hold it, so that the distant person could see their loved one in the bed. If prayer was requested, it seemed rather surreal to be praying for a person while holding the phone or tablet and trying to ensure the camera was pointing at the patient. These calls have been international on occasion, transmitted to the other side of the world.

On the occasions when there is conversation in a language other than English, the chaplain's role is to be present, to facilitate, to be a third party to what is going on. Being there when the distant person is saying their goodbyes, maybe thanking a parent for their life, is a privilege to observe but is naturally emotionally charged. All this happens while wearing full PPE, which is hot, and when the call drops off or technology fails it is frustrating. There is an awareness of the anxiety of the people waiting, distant, feeling powerless to re-establish that call, that vital link.

What of the future? Many routine activities we are used to are now missing. What is the new normal? We say we don't like routine, but many miss it. The hospital is slowly reverting back to its pre-crisis orientation, but there are hidden victims of this crisis: those who have not had their operations; those afraid to go to the GP and have missed an early diagnosis of a potentially fatal but treatable illness. Anxiety takes its toll on the mental health of hospital staff, and will continue to do so. Teams have been separated and individuals re-deployed. Wards have been moved and re-designated. Staff have encountered new colleagues. Many have been working in new and challenging situations. These are all potential disruptions which are not necessarily welcome. As teams reform, some fallout in terms of staff wellbeing has become noticeable.

## "an effective presence ... a mostly silent one"

Jan reports on her experience and reflections:

One impact of the virus was a sense of concerned unease that the chaplains' restricted movement around the hospital might change the perception, particularly that of staff, that we were not as available as we would normally be. General ward visiting was no longer a usual everyday event, and social distancing as well as other demands on staff time meant that normal conversations were less relaxed and frequent. How might we maintain our sense of availability for support under these circumstances?

I compared this sense of restriction and enforced lack of presence to a hospital scenario a few years back, when there had been a sudden death on hospital grounds involving a motor vehicle, with staff walking into work as the incident unfolded in front of them. Within hours, a large group meeting was arranged for distressed staff and there was space for them to talk about the impact this event had had. As a chaplain, I attended and mostly listened. Despite a sense of my own complete inadequacy as an effective presence, I afterwards received feedback about how one member of staff had made positive comments about a chaplain being a presence in that meeting, if a mostly silent one. Now because of the virus we couldn't repeat that sense of being physically present in the same way, so we have had to rely more, but not exclusively, on staff remembering that we are available, if only via the telephone. But how to remind them and how confident could we be of our usefulness?

As we were directed to socially distance by having our chaplaincy team office presence in the hospital reduced by fifty per cent, my own sense was one of dislocation and ineffectiveness, as new support groups in the hospital rapidly formed and publicized their availability for staff and bereaved relatives. But didn't we as chaplains already do this work each and every day? I wanted to document this twin sense of, on one hand, not physically being alongside staff and patients because of the virus restrictions and on the other hand, the internal concern about not being a "good enough" chaplain because this work is our natural remit and it felt disconcerting to not be able to carry it out fully when new groups were busy offering support. This sense of frustration about new support groups growing rapidly and yet not at the same time fully acknowledging an existing chaplaincy presence was echoed by fellow chaplains from other Trusts.

All in all, this has proved to be probably the most unsettling time in the last decade for our department. But a thought that sustained me personally was the advice to "watch and wait" for how we might be used in the future. A fellow chaplain suggested that when the worst of the pandemic had passed, we would then be needed to support those staff who had been traumatized by the nature and demands of the work, but might only feel ready to come and be supported once the immense pressure of virus-related work was reduced. We are noticing that this is starting to happen slowly in the weeks following the diminishing number of COVID-19 in-patients. As pressure gradually slackens, there is an unfolding of the full impact of the challenges to healthcare professionals, which is now becoming more visible, and staff are more likely to feel able to ask for help.

Just as importantly, as we continue to experience a year identified by a starkly changing COVID-19 landscape, the unwelcome and uncomfortable sense of dislocation for me has changed to one of curiosity and even a little excitement about how we might do things differently in the light of all that the pandemic is teaching us. It is important for us as chaplains and practical theologians to examine the effects of changes in the way we work and the new ways of being alongside that we have discovered through the necessity of social distancing and infection control. It feels as if we might have carried on doing the same thing in the same way had we not been challenged to develop differently for a post-pandemic world. There is no doubt that it has helped us to learn to live more comfortably with uncertainty.

## A road, "the one less travelled by" (Frost 2017: 7)

Sacha reports on his experience and reflections:

Within hours of the first lockdown, the main entrance to the hospital felt as if no one was in the building, perhaps a very quiet weekend or hot Bank Holiday. Empty wards, quiet corridors, red "no entry" signs and crosses of yellow and black tape across doors as if hiding a crime scene made walking around the hospital feel as if I was, at best, not required and at worst, singularly not welcome. It was as though I had stumbled into a nightmare, some other world, a different level of existence, where everything had a certain familiarity yet I was unable to connect or engage with anyone or anything that was happening. I sat bewildered in our department and felt that over ten years of chaplaincy had suddenly changed, and I had no idea what I should, or could, actually do. The hospital had changed from being a vast city, with bustling shops and coffee bars, corridors full of chattering people, staff walking swiftly from place to place, trolleys of equipment, patients in beds, trolleys, wheelchairs, out-patients clutching appointment letters, visitors carrying tea and newspapers to the wards... to a twenty-first-century brick-built Marie Celeste. It was as if everyone, and everything, was holding their breath, even the walls themselves. Perhaps that is exactly what was happening, with the then little understood coronavirus COVID-19 in the air.

Having practised healthcare chaplaincy as a relational ministry, where wandering the corridors, wards and units is the most normal thing to do, with chance encounters with patients, staff and visitors, and to be called to any urgent need at a bleep, it was now as if my most natural practice had been shredded, filed, no longer required. Our department offices were now also silent, with the usual team of volunteer pastoral visitors stood down, and four chaplains looking at each other as if we had all come in to cover the weekend together (when it would usually be just one of us) or perhaps as if waiting for an update following a major incident.

From evolving government guidelines and developing hospital practice, just as it was for everyone, rules and advice changed daily. The frequent moving of the wards and staff meant the need for awareness of how many COVID-19 patients were in the building, and which wards were green, amber or red; there was the sense of being constantly alert to minute-by-minute change. It meant learning how to navigate, pause and re-assess, re-orientate and re-trace steps from a ward that one could visit without PPE yesterday but where today it had become plastered with colours and signs shouting "No entry!" This early experience of a hospital working so very hard to prepare, re-assess and adjust operationally according to need, felt like an attempt to hold onto a ship in a storm without really being aware of which way the wind was blowing.

This tested even those of us who claim that "change and challenge" is our bread and butter! We felt we did not know where to go, or which wards/units we could visit, devoid of our usual wanderings and chance encounters and somewhat held at a distance. This was, of course, a sign of our own sense of deficiency, our sense of moral injury. This term emerged quickly in the COVID-19 literature in March 2020 because of the sudden and unexpected, unprecedented nature of the coronavirus outbreak. Originally used to describe the effect of conflict, it describes people's experience when feeling inadequate either through being underused or else expected to do something for which they may feel unprepared (Greene, Bloomfield and Billings 2020: 1). As a profession, which we claim is a paradigm of the contextual dialogue of narrative and praxis (Graham 2005, 2012), we reflected that we felt out of context, no longer part of the story and unable to practise.

Yet, this acknowledgement was the first step in recognizing our particular place in the COVID-19 story. Not only was this happening to us but to every single healthcare professional who themselves felt they were on the back foot and rushing to catch up with events and change that had reached exceptional heights. Like other hospital practitioners, we had to develop our practice, learn how to do things differently, learn from our experience and respond to the new context. This connects with the "challenge of double reflexivity" (Osmer 2008: 240), as outlined in Chapter 2, where both those involved in the story, or pastoral encounter, are changed.

Quite literally, thank God for practical theology where we feel our story and the story of those around us is worth hearing and sharing, where we are accompanied and in conversation, where we learn and develop together. It is a journey on a road, "the one less travelled by" (Frost 2017: 7), but it is an accompanied journey.

Thus far, in our shared reflections on "living with a virus", we have recalled our experiences of walking alongside the healthcare staff involved here. We have shared the times we have felt paralysed by not feeling part of the story, unable to practise or feeling inadequate, and yet increasingly the times when we have been right in the middle of the red-zone COVID-19 mess. We have shared our learning from the innumerable pastoral encounters with staff, patients and wayfarers, both physically and remotely, during the changing, challenging voyage of this pandemic. Demonstrating how practical theology is not only our life but is also a means of decision-making, for example in terms of faith care practice, we have shown how "living with a virus" further reveals the practical theology of healthcare chaplaincy. Just as poignantly as sharing the reflections of healthcare staff on the front line of COVID-19, we have also shared our reflections on some of our own experiences, personally and professionally, over this pandemic year.

We move now to offer our further reflections on the way in which our story has "created space" for us to build on reflective practice, which is the key tool of practical theology, looking back and looking forward. Opening the door to our discoveries, we also show the way in which others have shared with us their learning while alongside us, and we consider the possibilities of the path ahead, both for ourselves and in the hope that we may inspire those who work in any form of pastoral care, or the caring professions, or who may be able to use reflective practice as a tool for "creating space" for learning.

CHAPTER 10

# Looking back and looking forward

In taking time to pause and to reflect on over ten years of healthcare chaplaincy, we have "created space" to learn from our experiences in context and demonstrate how our story and practice have evolved. We have taken the opportunity to share our discoveries, plotting the course of that evolution. This began in the early chapters with looking through the lens of our own professional background, then our perception of the unique chaplain. We have outlined our understanding and model of practical theology and the reflective practice tool for learning. We have shown how our developments are mirrored in and outside the hospital context. This is a process of *looking back*, reflecting on these experiences and identifying our learning, pausing to share our discoveries, enabling us to reveal our adventure for learning. Now we will explore in different ways what we have gained by journeying through this storytelling reflective process. We will then *look forward* to where the path may next take us. We invite fellow practitioners to be inspired by our discoveries to "create space" to explore their own.

## Creating Space: room for reflection

Before drawing any further reflections on how far we have come, we pause here to consider how actually the whole *Creating Space* story is itself an example of reflective practice, used in practical theology, where learning from experience means the story is told and explored, and the continuous learning discerned. We will show how we have further built on theories, as mentioned in Chapter 3, of the experiential learning and reflective processes (Dewey 1933, 1938; Schön 1983; Kolb 1984; Rolfe

2014; Pearce 2018). Developing further Sacha's own research (Pearce 2018), we recognize that our story of *Creating Space* adds to his reflective work in healthcare and takes it beyond the hospital walls. Developing a culture of daily reflection, on any part of the chaplain's experience, provides an adventurous source for learning. We now outline in more detail these theories and developments as the building of our reflective process.

Being engaged with exploring an experience is an "interaction" between both the self and the surroundings (Dewey 1938: 42), and both are changed. As one discovery leads to another, "reflective thought is a chain" (Dewey 1933: 5) and seeks further learning. There is "continuity and interaction" and learning continues (Dewey 1938: 44). This is using "reflection-in-action", meaning to learn from the immediate experience (Schön 1983: 54), where the practitioner "re-frames" or sees from another perspective (Schön 1983: 131), developing learning in the light of previous experience yet still "unique" to the current situation (Schön 1983: 137). This means having "a reflective conversation with the situation" (Schön 1983: 163). It can mean "learning as a continuous, lifelong process" (Kolb 1984: 33), with a fluidity of learning rather than solution-finding, where learning is "the process whereby knowledge is created through the transformation of experience" (Kolb 1984: 41). Seeing experiential learning as a lifelong tool, Kolb argues that "integrative development" is a challenging yet fulfilling element of such a learning process (Kolb 1984: 209). This means being able to combine and sustain personal development in one's own work and use integrity as a wider, deeper and truthful sense of self-knowledge. The purpose of the latter, argues Kolb, is "to stand at the interface between social knowledge and the ever-novel predicaments and dilemmas we find ourselves in . . . to guide us through" and even contribute to the learning of others (Kolb 1984: 225). This sense of lifelong experiential learning involves "reflective thinking . . . with the curiosity and speculation that arise" (Rolfe 2014: 1183). This is "not to answer questions, but simply to raise them and to provoke responses through dialogue" (Rolfe 2014: 1183).

Developing both the work of Kolb (1984) and Rolfe (2014), Sacha's research project built on these areas of experiential learning and reflective processes. Following Kolb's view of the learning process as combining work and personal development, Sacha's project was developed using a reflective process for healthcare professionals at work, not for their professional development, but in order that they may nurture their wellbeing in their context. It involves both their knowledge of their experiences and a growing sense of self-awareness, building on the juxtaposition of Kolb's work on development and personal integrity. This further developed Kolb's application by using Sacha's own unique HELP Wellbeing Reflection Cycle. This has a useful acronym in a memorable four-stage model. It also uses questions at each stage that specifically invite self-awareness in the process of nurturing wellbeing through reflection-in-action. For Kolb and his predecessors, the fourth stage in a reflective cycle involves action to test out new learning. However, the HELP Wellbeing Reflection Cycle develops this stage as a platform for leaving the reflective space empowered, able to return to the workplace, with a greater sense of wellbeing. The new learning, the pondering, is not a solution but an ability to make an empowered step for personal and professional wellbeing, rather than leading to any conclusion that cognitively tests new knowledge. Sacha's doctoral thesis title includes the phrase "Building Space", referring not only to the architecture of the account of his research, but to the space created both within and among those who regularly reflect together before returning refreshed to the path.

To limit reflection to a one-off event could mean one finite piece of learning or defined solution after the event. Sacha's research project adds to Rolfe's work on healthcare professionals' practice by developing the healthcare culture of reflective practice with a simple, regular tool for informal dialogue and shared learning to nurture wellbeing. It facilitates "reflection-in-action", spontaneous reflection "on this situation now", in the daily work environment. His work, building on both Kolb and Rolfe, means "creating space" using his HELP cycle and nurturing regular, accessible use of reflection in healthcare with and beyond staff, as a foundation for volunteers, students, parishioners and an ever-growing constituency. "Creating Space" began with this new reflective process, but we show that this is both a tool for discovery and a feature of our journey, and now turn to consider further its role for others.

## Creating Space: space for others

We have shown previously the way in which we have "created space" for staff to reflect both within and outside the pandemic experience. We have demonstrated how we have "created space" for the learning and discoveries of our own pastoral care team and indeed regional colleagues in our chaplaincy conferences. Moreover, it has become a gratifying and important part of our departmental evolution to share our training, initially reserved for hospital pastoral visiting teams, with candidates from a much wider variety of settings. Over the last five years, we have been approached by hospital-based palliative care staff, volunteers planning to offer pastoral care in residential and nursing homes, and counselling and psychotherapy undergraduates as well as parish-based pastoral visitors and clergy. The feedback we received from a parish-based lay minister who had attended our training course was encouraging and suggested that we were touching something different from other training they had previously received. This candidate noted:

> The course put into words the way that I had approached previous pastoral encounters as a minister. I had struggled to identify with some ways/models offered by others in my early training as a Reader. When I began the training at Derriford, it was like a deep affirmation, a Big Yes, this is it, and I continue to be empowered to apply all I learnt in every pastoral encounter within my ministry and life; to have no religious agenda, to listen and to be deeply happy to leave the encounter with loose ends, to reflect and to pray in private and let go. Liberating, inclusive, joyful; challenging, deeply moving. In a ministry setting, I am free to be me and come alongside all God's children.

A priest who attended our most recent training group just before the start of the COVID-19 pandemic noted some months afterwards that:

> the course proved to be timely in some ways as I have found people feeling isolated or stressed are needing to talk. What

would normally be a ten-minute encounter on the phone or in the street easily becomes an hour as people find someone to listen.

The same priest gave us some encouraging feedback on our teaching of reflective practice, which of course forms a significant part of the training, and so we discovered that our training might be used by external training candidates, not only to improve pastoral listening but to offer reflective practice for groups in their own particular settings. He hit upon the idea of offering reflective practice to support teachers in his local Church of England primary school and subsequently relayed to us that the idea was indeed well received and supported by the school, despite the fact that the pandemic delayed its inception.

More recently, in 2021, it is rewarding to report that our pastoral training has now become part of ministerial and lay development offered through, and endorsed by, the Diocese of Exeter, where both clergy and laity can access the course either in person or remotely. Our current incarnation of a training course that incorporates candidates from a variety of settings (parish pastoral groups, university students, hospital volunteers and staff, clergy and lay ministers) means that learning takes place across contexts, enabling candidates to learn not just from the trainers but from each other through reflection in action learning groups.

Further work in this direction could also include the provision of a more fully focussed training on facilitating reflective practice for those who head up pastoral visitor groups in their parish or organization. Simply to train individuals for visiting in different pastoral teams and then offer nothing further would be to neglect the critical place of reflective practice in helping teams to grow from each other's experience in their pastoral work. We have emphasized this when, in the past, groups from mixed contexts have trained together with us and we have encouraged them to return to their parishes and ask for reflective practice from their pastoral leader or priest. This now needs to be made more formal for the growth, support and wellbeing of the pastoral visitors themselves, and in recognition of the demands of this kind of work. This, of course, may also link with clergy becoming more appreciative of, and comfortable with, reflective practice for their own wellbeing, which feeds into the concern that clergy are often reluctant to engage in this process for their own benefit, as well as for the benefit of those they manage or for whom they care professionally. We consider now what may be our own "next step".

## Creating Space: the next step

An ongoing journey of discovery, "Creating Space" is both our everyday "bread and butter" now and the source of nourishment in the future. Everywhere, and with everyone with whom we have been or are involved, we consider what "creating space" could mean to them in the future of their own journey and discoveries. We feel passionate about empowering others to find the richness of what they have discovered in their own context. Just as our own team of pastoral visitors describes the privilege of their work here and all that they are encouraged to learn through each pastoral encounter, so we offer our story inviting others to explore developing a similar "adventure for learning" paradigm in their own context.

As has been mentioned, one of our key hopes is the development of reflective practice in the parish, or elsewhere, following our training with those working in pastoral care. We have described our support of healthcare staff working in the COVID-19 pandemic and the way in which one-to-one pastoral encounters with staff and the "Space for Wellbeing" reflective groups have developed. The next step is to continue this across the hospital and nurture the use of "reflection for wellbeing" as a self-supporting tool for healthcare teams, both clinical and non-clinical. We are also developing support especially for nurses who are following the NHS "staff advocacy" model, learning how to support each other, but using our reflective model to complement their NHS "listening skills" training in this area.

As we anticipate additional next steps, these include plans for remote access to our pastoral training, which would likely not have taken place had it not been for the restrictions brought about by the pandemic. In March 2020, we had almost completed training for a cohort of candidates when we were forced to terminate live sessions because of impending lockdown. With no imminent possibility of seeing our pastoral volunteers return to the hospital, we had little option but to watch and wait, rather than rush into a new venture. In that time, across the globe, our means of communication, whether that be meetings, socializing, worship or training, have been completely revolutionized, and many of us have now experienced the advantages and the new normal of connecting through technology. The watching and waiting, as well as our increasing familiarity with the technology from using it for other purposes, was an important part of this process. Whilst it might have been unthinkable a year ago to try and conduct training in pastoral skills across a computer screen, that very idea has become a new possibility, and not simply to "get over" the problem of being unable to meet in person. Even when the pandemic has subsided, this medium creates new possibilities for those who might struggle to travel to attend live training. Now with the advantages of systems that allow not only whole-group teaching but the creation of effective breakout rooms for small group discussion, we can create our action learning groups once again. Unexpectedly, access to our training, especially for those who live in remote parts of Devon and Cornwall (indeed, anywhere else in the world) is a real possibility. Only a year ago, this opportunity for opening out our training to people over a wide geographical area would simply not have occurred to us and yet writing about it now in 2021, the idea seems like a completely natural next step, such is the impact of the pandemic and the growing popularity of available technology that makes this possible.

Another new step we want to encourage is for more chaplains to explore this material, considering how our story may help them learn more from their own narrative. We would urge chaplains to continue not only to use reflection in their own team but to demonstrate these skills to a wider audience. This too we hope to encourage in parish clergy, lay ministers and parish groups, to become more aware of and at ease with using reflective practice, self-awareness, learning together from experience, as a more common currency for discovery. Our hope too is to encourage pastoral care as more of a "being" ministry (Stobert 2020: 77), "being with" (Wells 2017: 7) and in so doing nurture within themselves and their team a willingness to be open, creating space for themselves, to discover more, for the adventure of learning.

## Creating Space: our story

In Chapter 1, both authors set out their own particular and quite different journeys into chaplaincy from previous careers. Here we both comment on those journeys from a much later stage in our ministries, as we look back and reflect on what chaplaincy means as our identity, how we have learnt from experience and what we have gained personally from this reflective work together and separately.

### Chaplain: priest and therapist (Jan)

Prior to ordination, and despite my own uncertainties, I felt called into a kind of ministry that would take and use my counselling training and experience from an existing occupation. The account of that journey in Chapter 1 highlighted the difficulty that the Church of England had in addressing a different kind of call since discernment of ministry was at the time, and still largely is, confined to historical, parish-based parameters. Therefore, even if such a vocational call was genuine, the Church was unable to respond appropriately, and it was challenging and often distressing to remain committed to believing in it. Thankfully, this call was eventually affirmed and is part and parcel of my identity as chaplain, priest and therapist. It appears very clear now, after some years as a chaplain, that my experience as a therapist cannot be partitioned or excluded from who I am as a chaplain. But what has chaplaincy done to my view of ministry?

It has highlighted for me the poignancy and reality of the God who is alongside; the God who is to be found in the strangest and most unpromising places we encounter in the hospital. It has alerted me to the possibilities that although we may create space, what fills that space is not ours to deliver, control or manipulate. There is a profound sense that we may be used as agents of possibility, of people being encouraged to tell their story, or being given room to simply "be". We mirror this notion of simply "being" for the patient also to "be", by allowing ourselves to "be" rather than focus on what we can "do". It is a matter of deep trust that we enter the vulnerable place of simply "showing up", rather than embodying someone who "fixes" or finds solutions, which tends to disempower those to whom we minister. For some, this may sound far too passive, but it is actually demanding work, and is an active and willing participation in the story unfolding in front of us without being intrusive or manipulative. If we are willing to "be", rather than simply "do", then we are more likely to be open to discover God's presence in the stories of those we encounter, in the faces of those who come to us for help, but who often happen to be those who teach us the most. This notion is much more eloquently expressed in Sam Wells' insistence that "with" is the most important word in the Christian faith (Wells 2017: 7). He maintains that "chaplaincy is precisely about showing up and hanging about in places where transformation happens" and "seeking to be present, intentionally" (Wells 2017: 118). It is also encapsulated in Henri Nouwen's writing on hospitality:

> Hospitality, therefore, means primarily the creation of a free space where the stranger can enter and become a friend instead of an enemy. Hospitality is not to change people, but to offer them space where change can take place. It is not to bring men and women over to our side, but to offer freedom not disturbed by dividing lines. It is not to lead our neighbour into a corner where there are no alternatives left, but to open a wide spectrum of options for choice and commitment. It is not an educated intimidation with good books, good stories and good works, but the liberation of fearful hearts so that words can find roots and bear ample fruit. It is not a method of making our God and our way into the criteria of happiness, but the opening of an opportunity to others to find their God and their way. The paradox of hospitality is that it wants to create emptiness, not a fearful emptiness, but a friendly emptiness where strangers can enter and discover themselves as created free; free to sing their own songs, speak their own languages, dance their own dances; free also to leave and follow their own vocations. Hospitality is not a subtle invitation to adopt the lifestyle of the host, but the gift of a chance for the guest to find his own (Nouwen 1998: 49).

Of course, there are times when we are required to be more proactive, for example when we are called out in the middle of the night or at end of life, when there is often a desire in patients or relatives for us to "do something religious". Nevertheless, what we do is to gently assist them in finding appropriate ways to care and minister to those in need, which may or may not include offering prayers. Above all, however, the most important thing we can do is to *be with* them at this crucial moment; that is by far the priority over any words (liturgy or otherwise) that we might speak. In all of this, as we accompany them on a difficult journey, we are aware of being accompanied ourselves by a God who is alongside and strengthens us when we feel most inadequate; we are only able to offer a steadying presence by realizing we too are strengthened and steadied by knowing that God is with us.

As we have previously noted, chaplaincy is edgy and messy, for which, with hindsight, I am deeply grateful. The messiness is cleverly disguised as an invaluable teacher and has put into perspective my fears about "getting things right", particularly with regard to worship—an unfortunate hangover from my parish curacy, where liturgical exactitude was a source of anxiety. Chaplaincy, particularly in the mental health setting where I continue to work in addition to the hospital, has been a place of surprise and unpredictability, where patients have taught me that I need to be flexible and prioritize listening and accompanying, rather than worrying about perfecting worship or always getting things right. Each visit afresh, I need to learn what they are teaching me as I quietly loiter in their communal space, rather than stride in and assume I have something to deliver whether or not they want it. This is especially true for mental health settings, but it is vital learning in all kinds of places, where we need to practise quiet, attentive sitting and not rush in to feverishly minister and do all kinds of religious things. Some days in the unit, a good number of patients want to have conversations with us, and other days we are far less in demand. Nevertheless, we "show up" and make ourselves available, although that is not always a comfortable place to inhabit for those feeling and needing to be busy, engaged and useful.

This learning is not solely and exclusively relevant for chaplains. Both of us attest to the idea that chaplaincy ministry has considerably changed our way of being in any other ministry setting, such as parish life, to which we both contribute from time to time. Allowing ourselves to sit in the place where there are no expectations of the nature of our ministry, but rather being open and receptive to the needs of whoever is in front of us, is no less vital to ministry outside of chaplaincy.

## Chaplain: priest and reflective practitioner (Sacha)

From long before dawn on the day of my first ordination, now twenty years ago, I knew that I was stepping out on the journey of the evolving "me", and into a deepening awareness that I had so much more to discover, to learn and become. Each step is far more than travelling but is inner journeying by "tracing the sacred" and exploring "the hermeneutics of lived religion by wandering its uncharted and changing territory" (Ganzevoort 2009: 6). Standing in the south aisle of Salisbury Cathedral, with my white stole over my left arm, as the procession began, I stepped into my life. From deacon and curate to priest and rural parish incumbent, to hospital chaplain, I have continued to be and am always becoming, in the words of St Irenaeus, "fully alive".

"All things came into being through him," says the author of St John's Prologue (John 1:3), as he weaves an image of life with change as its very essence. It is life being nurtured from darkness to light, from functional to organic, from nothingness to fulfilment, indeed from humanity to divinity. It is an image of life coming into its fullness through revelation of the presence of the incarnate divine, woven deep within human experience. To "come into being" means to grow as a whole person. It is to discover our true selves, how we grow to our fullest potential, into who we really are, into whom God has called us to become. It is this journey of discovery, this vocation to be fully whoever it is that I am, that inspires my yearning to nurture that self-awareness in others.

Rowan Williams described vocation as "God's summons into existence itself" as each of us is called to nurture the development of the whole person: "Only when I am conscious of being called by God to be myself in Christ can I find what specific work He asks of me in passing on that discovery and that hope to others" (Williams 2001: 92). "To be myself in Christ" means to discover self-awareness through reflection and reflexivity and identify how to fulfil my potential. This also continues to energize my desire to empower others to self-discover, the nurturing of which is at the very heart of learning through human experience.

The "coming home" to practical theology and healthcare chaplaincy was another step on my journey of "life in its fullness", stepping into the wilderness with the incarnational God of Bethlehem's animal cave, Jerusalem's Golgotha, the Galilean lakeside breakfast and the Emmaus Road. The contextual theology of learning through our grubby, earthy reality of acute human experience is, for me, other words for saying I continue to learn, I believe, that I am called to the "being" of the practical theology of healthcare chaplaincy.

Our lives are given credibility and connection by telling our stories of human experience (Bochner and Riggs 2014; Swinton 2015), so another part of my story is my deeper learning by researching the tool of reflective practice, which after all means "learning from experience". Now, alongside my fine colleague, telling our story of *Creating Space* is another step on my own evolving journey as we learn more and share our discoveries.

It is this continued openness, a willingness to "be" and to "become", to continuously learn, that is the richness of "being fully alive". It is each pastoral encounter, each place of "mutual hospitality" (Walton, M. 2012: 226), each "blurred encounter" (Reader and Baker 2009) where being "empty handed" (Swift 2009: 175) holds the experiences of the storyteller, that also makes me "fully alive". It is in the gift that each storyteller gives me, in trusting me with their heartfelt, often until now untold story, that tells me that as a chaplain I am "tracing the sacred" (Ganzevoort 2009: 6), and therefore standing on whatever may be the storyteller's holy ground.

### Creating Space: your story?

*Creating Space: Story, Reflection and Practice in Healthcare Chaplaincy* is *our* story, our journey of discovery. This we have revealed by showing that practical theology is our reflective life, our practice, and so it is our means of exploring, discovery and learning. This we do by "creating space", a ministry of "being with", whether with patients, staff or accompanying anyone, as well as "being with" each other as colleagues. We "create space" with "empty hands", with the "mutual hospitality" of the "welcoming guest". Perhaps our final thought, or current conclusion, would be this invitation, as we open the doors of our discovery to share them with you: "How will *you* use *our* story to create space in your own context to explore your own story and practice?" Happy journeying!

# Bibliography

Adie, K. (2002), *The Kindness of Strangers: The Autobiography*, London: Hodder & Stoughton.
Archbishops' Council (2000), *Common Worship: Services and Prayers for the Church of England*, London: Church House Publishing.
Aull Davies, C. (2008), *Reflexive Ethnography: A Guide to Researching Selves and Others*, 2nd edn, Abingdon, United Kingdom: Routledge.
Baxendale, R. (2015), "Observing, Recording and Analysing Spiritual Care in an Acute Setting", in J. Pye, P. Sedgewick, and A. Todd (eds), *Critical Care: Delivering Spiritual Care in Healthcare Contexts*, London: Jessica Kingsley Publishers, pp. 185–204.
Billings, A. (2004), *Secular Lives, Sacred Hearts*, London: SPCK.
Bochner, A. and Riggs, N. (2014), "Practising Narrative Inquiry", in P. Leavy (ed.), *The Oxford Handbook of Qualitative Research*, Oxford: Blackwell Publishers, pp. 195–222.
Bolton, G. (2010), *Reflective Practice, Writing and Professional Development (3rd edn)*, London: SAGE Publications.
Bombeck, E. (1978), *If Life is a Bowl of Cherries, What am I Doing in the Pits?* New York: McGraw-Hill.
Braun, V. and Clarke, V. (2006), "Using thematic analysis in psychology", *Qualitative Research in Psychology* 3:2, pp. 77–101.
Bulman, C. and Schutz, S. (eds), (2008), *Reflective Practice in Nursing* (4th edn), Oxford: Blackwell Publishing Ltd.
Bushell, S. (2008), "The Craft of Spiritual Care", *The Journal of Health Care Chaplaincy* 9:1/2, pp. 57–60.
Cameron, H., Bhatti, D., Duce, C., Sweeney, J. and Watkins, C. (2010), *Talking about God in Practice: Theological Action Research and Practical Theology*, London: SCM Press.

Caperon, J., Todd, A. and Walters, J. (eds), (2017), *A Christian Theology of Chaplaincy*, London: Jessica Kingsley Publishers.

Child, L. (1997), *Killing Floor*, London: Bantam Press.

Church of England (2020), Qualities for Discernment. Priest and Distinctive Deacon, <https://www.churchofengland.org/life-events/vocations>, accessed via hard copy from Diocese of Exeter, May 2021.

Church Times, General Synod Report, 1 March 2019, <https://www.churchtimes.co.uk/articles/2019/1-march/news/uk/general-synod-unease-on-new-opt-out-rules-on-deanery-terms>, accessed 2 July 2021.

Cobb, M. (2005), *The Hospital Chaplain's Handbook: A Guide for Good Practice*, Norwich: Canterbury Press.

Cobb, M., Swift, C. and Todd, A. (2015), "Introduction to Chaplaincy Studies", in C. Swift, M. Cobb and A. Todd (eds), *A Handbook of Chaplaincy Studies: Understanding Spiritual Care in Public Places*, Abingdon: Routledge, pp. 1–9.

de Vries, R., Berlinger, N. and Cadge, W. (2008), *Lost in Translation: The Chaplain's Role in Healthcare*, The Hastings Center Report 2008 Nov/Dec; 38(6), pp. 23–7.

de Waal, E. (2003), *Living with Contradiction: Benedictine Wisdom for Everyday Living, Volume 3*, Norwich: Canterbury Press.

Department of Pastoral and Spiritual Care, Derriford Hospital (2016), *Creating Space: The Pastoral Encounter*, unpublished.

Derrida, J. and Dufourmantelle, A. (2000), *Of Hospitality. Anne Dufourmantelle invites Jacques Derrida to respond*, tr. R. Bowlby, Stanford, CA: Stanford University Press.

Dewey, J. (1933), *How We Think*, Boston, MA: DC Heath and Co.

Dewey, J. (1938), *Experience and Education*, New York, NY: Simon and Schuster.

Diocese of Peterborough, <https://www.peterborough-diocese.org.uk/ordained-ministry/what-does-ordained-ministry-look-like>, accessed 2 July 2021.

Eliot, T. S. (1944), *Four Quartets*, London: Faber and Faber.

Emerson, R., Fretz, R. and Shaw, L. (2011), *Writing Ethnographic Fieldnotes*, 2nd edn, Chicago, IL: University of Chicago Press.

Fielding, N. (2008), "Ethnography", in N. Gilbert (ed.), *Researching Social Life*, London: SAGE, pp. 266–84.
Fitchett, G. and Nolan, S. (2015), *Spiritual Care in Practice*, London: Jessica Kingsley Publishers.
Frost, R. (2017), *Mountain Interval*, New York: Henry Holt.
Ganzevoort, R. (2009), "Forks in the Road when Tracing the Sacred, Practical Theology as Hermeneutics of Lived Religion", Presidential Address, International Academy of Practical Theology, Chicago, IL, 3 August 2009.
Gibbs, G., Farmer, B. and Eastcott, D. (1988), *Learning by Doing. A Guide to teaching and learning methods. FEU: Birmingham Polytechnic.*
Gilliat-Ray, S. and Arshad, M. (2015), "Multifaith Working", in C. Swift, M. Cobb and A. Todd (eds), *A Handbook of Chaplaincy Studies: Understanding Spiritual Care in Public Places*, Abingdon: Routledge, pp. 109–19.
Graham, E. (2009), *Words Made Flesh: Writings in Pastoral and Practical Theology*, London: SCM Press.
Graham, E. (2011), "The 'virtuous circle', Religion and the practices of happiness", in J. Atherton, E. Graham and I. Steedman (eds), *The Practices of Happiness: Political economy, religion and wellbeing*, Abingdon: Routledge, pp. 224–34.
Graham, E. (2012), "Feminist Theory", in B. Miller-McLemore (ed.), *The Wiley-Blackwell Companion to Practical Theology*, Chichester: Blackwell Publishing, pp. 193–203.
Graham, E. (2017), "The state of the art: Practical theology yesterday, today and tomorrow: New directions in practical theology", *Theology* 120:3 (2017), pp. 172–80.
Graham, E., Walton, H. and Ward, F. (2005), *Theological Reflection: Methods*, London: SCM Press.
Greene, T., Bloomfield, M. A. P. and Billings, J. (2020), "Psychological trauma and moral injury in religious leaders during COVID-19", *Psychological Trauma: Theory, Research, Practice, and Policy 12* (S1), S143–S145.

Groen, J. and Kawalilak, C. (2016), "Creating Spaces for Transformative Learning in the Workplace", *New Directions for Adult and Continued Education* 152 (2016), pp. 61–71.

Guba, E. and Lincoln, Y. (1994), "Competing Paradigms in Qualitative Research", in N. Denzin and Y. Lincoln (eds), *Handbook of Qualitative Research*, 1st edn, Thousand Oaks, CA: Sage, pp. 105–17.

Guite, M. (2012), *Sounding the Seasons: Seventy Sonnets for the Church Year*, Norwich: Canterbury Press.

Hammersley, M. and Atkinson, P. (2007), *Ethnography: Principles in Practice*, 3rd edn, Abingdon: Routledge.

Johns, C. (2009), *Becoming a Reflective Practitioner*, Chichester: Wiley-Blackwell.

Kelly, E. (2010), "Reflective Practice: Strategy, Structures and Significance", *Scottish Journal of Healthcare Chaplaincy*, pp. 48–51.

Kelly, E. (2012), "The Development of Healthcare Chaplaincy", *The Expository Times* 123:10, pp. 469–78.

Kelly, E. and Paterson, M. (2013), "Values-Based Reflective Practice", *Practical Theology* 6:1, pp. 51–68.

Kelly, E. and Swinton, J. (2020), *Chaplaincy and the Soul of Health and Social Care: Fostering Spiritual Wellbeing in Emerging Paradigms of Care*, London: Jessica Kingsley Publishers.

Kennedy, J. and Stirling, I. (2013), "Innovation in Spiritual Care", *The Scottish Journal of Healthcare Chaplaincy* 16 (special), pp. 62–3.

Kolb, D. (1984), *Experiential Learning: Experience as The Source of Learning and Development*, Upper Saddle River, NJ: Prentice Hall.

Lewis, C. S. (1942), *The Weight of Glory*, London: SPCK.

Lewis-Anthony, J. (2009), *If You Meet George Herbert on the Road ... Kill Him! Radically Re-Thinking Priestly Ministry*, London: Mowbray.

Long, A. (1990), *Listening*, London: Darton, Longman and Todd Ltd.

Mason, J. (2002), *Qualitative Researching*, London: Sage.

Mathews, G. and Izquierdo, C. (2009), *Pursuit of Happiness*, New York: Berghahn Books.

McClung, E., Grossoehme, D. and Jacobson, A. (2006), "Collaborating with Chaplains to Meet Spiritual Needs", *Medsurg Nursing* 15.3 (2006), pp. 147–56.

McNiff, J. (2013), *Action Research: Principles and Practice*, 3rd edn, Abingdon: Routledge.

Merriam-Webster Dictionary, "encounter", <https://www.merriam-webster.com/dictionary/encounter>, accessed 2 July 2021.

Merriam-Webster Dictionary, "hospitality", <https://www.merriam-webster.com/dictionary/hospitality>, accessed 2 July 2021.

Moody, C. (1999), "Spirituality and Sector Ministry", in G. Legood (ed.), *Chaplaincy: The Church's Sector Ministries*, New York, NY: Cassell, pp. 15–24.

Moon, J. (1999), *Reflection in Learning and Professional Development*, Abingdon: Routledge Falmer.

Mowat, H. (2008), *The Potential for Efficacy of Healthcare Chaplains and Spiritual Care Provision in the NHS (UK)*, NHS Yorkshire and Humber: Mowat Research.

Mowat, H., Bunniss, S., Snowden, A. and Wright, L. (2013), "Listening as health care", *The Scottish Journal of Healthcare Chaplaincy* 16 (special).

Mowat, H. and Swinton, J. (2007), *What do chaplains do? The role of the chaplain in meeting the spiritual needs of patients*, Aberdeen: Mowat Research.

Nouwen, H. (1979), *The Wounded Healer*, New York: Doubleday.

Nouwen, H. (1996), *Bread for the Journey*, London: Darton, Longman and Todd.

Nouwen, H. (1998), *Reaching Out*, London: Fount.

Nouwen, H., McNeill, D. and Morrison, D. (2008), *Compassion: A Reflection on the Christian Life*, London: Darton, Longman and Todd.

O'Laughlin, M. (2005), *Henri Nouwen: His Life and Vision*, New York, NY: Orbis.

O'Nuallain, F. (ed.) (2018), *The Kindness of Strangers: Travel Stories that Make your Heart Grow*, London: Summerdale Publishing Ltd.

Osmer, R. R. (2008), *Practical Theology: An Introduction*, Grand Rapids, MI: Wm. B. Eerdmans Publishing Co.

Paterson, M. (2015), "Supervision, Support and Safe Practice", in C. Swift, M. Cobb and A. Todd (eds), *A Handbook of Chaplaincy Studies*, Abingdon: Routledge, pp. 149–59.

Pattison, S. (2015a), "Situating Chaplaincy in the United Kingdom: The Acceptable Face of 'Religion'?", in C. Swift, M. Cobb and A. Todd (eds), *A Handbook of Chaplaincy Studies: Understanding Spiritual Care in Public Places*, Abingdon: Routledge, pp. 14–30.

Pattison, S. (2015b), "Chaplaincy as Public Theology: A Reflective Exploration", *Health and Social Care Chaplaincy* 3(2), pp. 110–28.

Pearce, S. J. T. (2018), "'Building Space: Developing Reflection for Wellbeing.' Can a chaplain help healthcare professionals develop reflective practice for wellbeing for themselves and their team?", Thesis. Doctor of Professional Studies in Practical Theology. University of Chester.

Pye, J., Sedgewick, P. and Todd, A. (eds) (2015), *Critical Care: Delivering Spiritual Care in Healthcare Contexts*, London: Jessica Kingsley Publishers.

Reader, J. and Baker, C. (2009), *Entering the New Theological Space: Blurred Encounters of Faith, Politics and Community*, Farnham: Ashgate.

Rogers, C. (1959), *A Theory of Therapy, Personality, and Interpersonal Relationships: As Developed in the Client-centered Framework*, New York: McGraw-Hill.

Rohr, R. (2011), *Falling Upward: A Spirituality For The Two Halves Of Life*, Hoboken: Wiley.

Rolfe, G. (2014), "Rethinking reflective education: What would Dewey have done?", *Nurse Education Today* 34 (2014), pp. 1179–83.

Schön, D. (1983), *The Reflective Practitioner: How Professionals Think in Action*, Farnham: Ashgate.

Slater, V. (2015), "Developing Practice-Based Evidence", in C. Swift, M. Cobb and A. Todd (eds), *Handbook of Chaplaincy Studies: Understanding Spiritual Care in Public Places*, Abingdon: Routledge, pp. 63–75.

Smith, M. and Puczko, L. (2017), "Introduction", in M. Smith and L. Puczko, *The Routledge Handbook of Health Tourism*, Abingdon: Routledge, pp. 1–5.

Speck, P. (1988), *Being There: Pastoral Care in Time of Illness*, London: SPCK.

Speck, P. (2010), "Spiritual/religious issues in care of the dying", in J. Ellershaw and S. Wilkinson (eds), *Care of the dying: a pathway to excellence*, 2nd edn, New York: Oxford University Press, pp. 90–105.

Stobert, M. (2020), "Healthcare Chaplaincy as Professional Artistry", in E. Kelly and J. Swinton (eds), *Chaplaincy and the Soul of Health and Social Care: Fostering Spiritual Wellbeing in Emerging Paradigms of Care*, London: Jessica Kingsley Publishers, pp. 62–80.

Stoddart, E. (2014), *Advancing Practical Theology: Critical Discipleship for Disturbing Times*, London: SCM Press.

Sturgis, P. (2008), "Designing Samples", in N. Gilbert (ed.), *Researching Social Life*, 3rd edn, London: SAGE, pp. 166–81.

Sullender, S. (2017), "Section Three. Reflecting on Practice. Editor's Introduction", *Reflective Practice: Formation and Supervision in Ministry* 37, pp. 105–6.

Swift, C. (2009), *Hospital Chaplaincy in the Twenty-first Century: The Crisis of Spiritual Care on the NHS*, Farnham: Ashgate Press.

Swift, C. (2015), "Health Care Chaplaincy", in C. Swift, M. Cobb and A. Todd (eds), *A Handbook of Chaplaincy Studies: Understanding Spiritual Care in Public Places*, Abingdon: Routledge, pp. 163–74.

Swift, C., Cobb, M. and Todd, A. (eds) (2015), *A Handbook of Chaplaincy Studies: Understanding Spiritual Care in Public Places*, Abingdon: Routledge.

Swinton, J. (2001), *Spirituality in Mental Health Care: Rediscovering a 'Forgotten' Dimension*, London: Jessica Kingsley Publishers.

Swinton, J. (2015), "Afterword", in G. Fitchett and S. Nolan (eds), *Spiritual Care in Practice*, London: Jessica Kingsley Publishers, pp. 299–305.

Swinton, J. and Kelly, E. (2015), "Contextual Issues: Health and Healing", in C. Swift, M. Cobb and A. Todd (eds), *A Handbook of Chaplaincy Studies: Understanding Spiritual Care in Public Places*, Abingdon: Routledge, pp. 175–85.

Swinton, J. and Mowat, H. (2006) *Practical Theology and Qualitative Research*, London: SCM Press.

Swinton, J. and Pattison, S. (2010), "Moving beyond clarity: towards a thin, vague, and useful understanding of spirituality in nursing care", *Nursing Philosophy* 11, pp. 226-37.

Swinton, J. and Vanderpot, L. (2017), "Religion and Spirituality in Nursing", in M. Balboni and J. Peteet (eds), *Spirituality and Religion Within the Culture of Medicine*, New York, NY: Oxford University Press, pp. 215-29.

Thornton, T. (2013), *Character and Charism—how can we shape the future?* Bishop of Truro's lecture to clergy and ordinands, College of St Mark and St John, Plymouth.

Timmins, F., Caldeira, S., Murphy, M., Pujol, N., Sheaf, G., Weathers, E. and Flanagan, B. (2017), "The Role of the Healthcare Chaplain: A Literature Review", *Journal of Healthcare Chaplaincy* 24 (3) pp. 87-106, <https://www.tandfonline.com/doi/full/10.1080/08854726.2017.1338048>, accessed 2 July 2021.

Todd, A. (2011, May), *Re-envisaging church in the light of current chaplaincy practice*. Paper presented at the Faith in Research Conference, London.

Todd, A., Cobb, M. and Swift, C. (2015), "Conclusion", in C. Swift, M. Cobb and A. Todd (eds), *A Handbook of Chaplaincy Studies: Understanding Spiritual Care in Public Places*, Abingdon: Routledge, pp. 327-35.

Walters, J. (2017), "Twenty-First Century Chaplaincy: Finding the Church in the Post Secular", in J. Caperon, A. Todd and J. Walters (eds), *A Christian Theology of Chaplaincy*, London: Jessica Kingsley Publishers, pp. 43-58.

Walton, H. (2002), "Speaking in Signs: Narrative and Trauma in Pastoral Theology", *Scottish Journal of Healthcare Chaplaincy* 5:2, pp. 2-5.

Walton, M. (2012), "The welcoming guest: Practices of mutual hospitality in Chaplaincy", in D. Louw, T. Ito and U. Elsdorfer (eds), *Encounter in Pastoral Care and Spiritual Healing*, Zurich: Lit Verlag, pp. 220-34.

Wells, S. (2017), *Incarnational Ministry: Being with the Church*, Norwich: Canterbury Press.

Whipp, M. (2017), "Embedding Chaplaincy: Integrity and Presence", in J. Caperon, A. Todd and J. Walters (eds), *A Christian Theology of Chaplaincy*, London: Jessica Kingsley Publishers, pp. 101–17.

Whorton, B. (2011), *Reflective Caring: Imaginative Listening to Pastoral Experience*, London: SPCK.

Williams, R. (2001), Appendix 5, Vocation. In *The Way Ahead: Church of England Schools in the New Millenium* (GS1406), London, United Kingdom: Church House Publishing.

Williams, T. (1957), *A Streetcar Named Desire*, London: Penguin.

EU GPSR Authorized Representative:

LOGOS EUROPE, 9 rue Nicolas Poussin, 17000 La Rochelle, France

contact@logoseurope.eu

www.ingramcontent.com/pod-product-compliance
Lightning Source LLC
Chambersburg PA
CBHW071424160426
43195CB00013B/1803